FLAT BELLY ANTI-INFLAMMATORY DIET FOR BEGINNERS

Simple and Affordable Tips to Reduce Bloating, Improve Gut Health, and Boost Longevity & Vitality

Dr. Amanda Borre, D.C.

TABLE OF CONTENTS

INTRODUCTION iv

CHAPTER 1
Understanding Inflammation and Its Impact 1

CHAPTER 2
Starting Your Anti-Inflammatory Journey 19

CHAPTER 3
Anti-Inflammatory Recipes for Beginners 37

CHAPTER 4
Meal Planning and Prep 57

CHAPTER 5
Beyond Diet—Lifestyle Factors Influencing Inflammation 77

CHAPTER 6
Overcoming Challenges and Staying Motivated 97

CHAPTER 7
Success Stories and Real-life Applications 113

CHAPTER 8
Advanced Topics in Anti-Inflammatory Practices 129

CONCLUSION 145

REFERENCES 149

INTRODUCTION

Nine years ago, my life changed dramatically. I remember waking up every morning feeling exhausted, despite a full night's sleep, and struggling with persistent pain and unpredictable digestive woes. As a healthcare professional, it was humbling to find myself at the mercy of my own body's inflammatory responses. It wasn't until I embraced an anti-inflammatory diet that I truly understood the profound impact food could have on my well-being. Within weeks, my energy returned, my pain diminished, and I felt revitalized—more in control of my health than ever before.

My name is Dr. Amanda Borre, D.C., and I have dedicated my career to guiding others toward achieving their best health. My journey into the world of anti-inflammatory eating wasn't just about personal relief; it sparked a passion to share this powerful tool with as many people as possible through my practice at Lifelong Metabolic Center. This book is an extension of that mission. It is crafted to demystify the principles of an anti-inflammatory diet and provide you, regardless of your cooking experience or budget, with the tools to integrate these principles into your daily life.

This guide is specifically designed for individuals who are navigating the complexities of maintaining health in today's world. Whether you are a Baby Boomer, a member of Generation X, or a Xennial, you will find that this book speaks directly to your unique needs and challenges. It is tailored to help you understand how inflammation affects your body and how you can counteract it with simple, delicious, and quick meal solutions.

In the following chapters, you will embark on a journey that begins with a deep dive into what inflammation is and how it impacts your body. From there, we will explore how to incorporate anti-inflammatory foods into your daily meals with ease. The book includes success stories from real people who have transformed their lives through similar changes, advanced topics for those who wish to deepen their understanding, and a special section dedicated to overcoming common hurdles.

I have ensured that every piece of advice is backed by scientific research and practical experience, making it not only educational but also actionable. You will find this book to be a blend of empathetic, positive, and supportive text, intended to encourage you every step of the way. Moreover, I have included prompts and questions to help you reflect on your own health and dietary habits, making your reading experience interactive and personally relevant.

As you turn each page, remember that every small change you make brings you closer to a more vibrant and healthier version of yourself. I am confident that with the insights and strategies outlined in this book, you can significantly enhance your health and vitality. Let's start this journey together, with hope and enthusiasm, towards a healthier, inflammation-free life.

CHAPTER 1
Understanding Inflammation and Its Impact

Have you ever wondered why your body reacts the way it does to a splinter in your finger or a sprained ankle? That redness, warmth, and swelling are your body's expert responders in action—it's inflammation working to protect and heal you. However, not all inflammation is fleeting or beneficial; sometimes, it overstays its welcome, becoming less of a hero and more of a lingering concern. In this chapter, we'll explore the nuanced roles of inflammation in your body, from its essential healing functions to its potential to disrupt your well-being when it becomes chronic. By grasping these concepts, you'll be better equipped to nurture your body's immune responses and foster long-term health through informed lifestyle choices.

1.1 What is Inflammation? A Simple Guide to Complex Biology

Inflammation is essentially your body's natural defense mechanism against injuries and infections. It's a critical part of the immune system's response, involving an array of cells and biological processes designed to protect and heal the body. When harmful bacteria invade or an injury occurs, your immune system dispatches an army of white blood cells to enclose and defeat the threat. This process increases blood flow to the affected area, which is why you might notice warmth and redness. Fluids carrying immune cells also accumulate, leading to swelling, while chemicals released by the white blood cells can stimulate nerve endings, causing pain.

These signs, while temporarily uncomfortable, are indicative of your body's healing forces at work. Redness and heat result from increased blood flow, which helps with the transport of immune cells and nutrients essential for repair. Swelling acts as a sort of isolation chamber, concentrating the immune response in the area that needs it most. Pain, though unpleasant, serves as a natural deterrent, discouraging you from using the affected part of your body and thus preventing further injury.

The benefits of inflammation are most apparent when it is acute—short-lived and directly related to tissue healing. This type of inflammation is vital; without it, injuries would not heal, and infections could become deadly. However, when inflammation becomes chronic, persisting beyond the healing process without a clear reason, it can lead to a myriad of health issues. Chronic inflammation can stealthily impact your body, contributing to the development of diseases such as arthritis, cardiovascular diseases, and even some forms of cancer.

This prolonged inflammatory response can often be silent, not showing the overt signs we associate with acute inflammation but quietly disrupting your body's internal balance and gradually degrading tissue.

Furthermore, systemic inflammation—that is, inflammation that occurs throughout the body—can have ripple effects on your overall health. It's not just about localized redness or swelling; it's about an ongoing, low-grade inflammatory response that can slowly compromise organ systems and metabolic functions. This type of inflammation can be influenced by numerous factors, including diet, lifestyle, and environmental exposures, which can all contribute to its persistence or management.

Understanding inflammation in its dual roles—as both protector and potential perpetrator—can empower you to make informed decisions about your health. Recognizing the signs and knowing when to seek help or how to adjust your lifestyle can make a significant difference in managing inflammation and maintaining a healthy, long, vibrant life. As we continue to explore inflammation's complexities, keep in mind that knowledge is not just power—it's prevention.

1.2 Chronic vs. Acute Inflammation: Knowing the Difference

Understanding the distinction between acute and chronic inflammation is crucial, as each affects your body differently and requires unique approaches to management. Acute inflammation is your body's immediate, short-term response to tissue injury or an invading pathogen. Picture this: you're cooking and accidentally slice your finger. Almost immediately, the area becomes red, warm, and swollen. This is acute inflammation springing into action, aiming to protect and heal the wound. It's a localized, intense response that typically resolves once the healing process is complete, usually within a few days to a week. This type of inflammation is essential—it's your body's frontline defense against infections and injuries, initiating repair and blocking further harm.

In contrast, chronic inflammation is a slower, more prolonged inflammatory response that can persist for months or even years. It's less about immediate survival and more about responding to prolonged threats to your health, such as persistent infections, prolonged exposure to irritants, or diseases like obesity. However, chronic inflammation often exists below the threshold of pain, meaning it can silently damage tissue over long periods without obvious symptoms. This type of inflammation is particularly insidious because it contributes to a host of non-communicable diseases, including some forms of cancer, heart disease, diabetes, and Alzheimer's disease. Unlike acute inflammation, which is visibly intense and beneficial, chronic inflammation often requires medical intervention to detect and manage.

Triggers for acute inflammation are typically immediate and clear, such as infections, injuries, or surgical interventions. Your body reacts swiftly to neutralize the threat and commence the healing process. Chronic inflammation, however, can be triggered by more subtle, ongoing factors. These include sustained stress, exposure to environmental pollutants, smoking, obesity, and even prolonged sedentary behavior. Each of these factors can subtly upregulate inflammatory processes in your body, often without clear symptoms, leading to gradual deterioration in tissue function and increased risk of chronic diseases.

Managing these two types of inflammation requires different strategies. Acute inflammation, being a necessary part of the healing process, often needs little more than basic first aid and proper hygiene to prevent infection. On the other hand, managing chronic inflammation often involves a more holistic approach. Lifestyle and dietary changes are pivotal—incorporating anti-inflammatory foods into your diet, increasing physical activity, reducing stress, and avoiding known inflammatory triggers like smoking and excessive alcohol consumption. For instance, integrating foods rich in omega-3 fatty acids, such as salmon and flaxseeds, can help regulate your body's inflammatory processes. Regular exercise not only helps in managing weight but also in promoting better circulation, which can help reduce inflammation levels throughout the body.

Moreover, understanding and addressing the underlying causes of chronic inflammation, such as obesity or stress, is essential for effective management. Medical interventions may also be necessary, especially when lifestyle changes alone do not sufficiently control the inflammatory response. In such cases, healthcare professionals might recommend therapeutic strategies, including medications designed to target specific inflammatory pathways, guided by detailed health evaluations and ongoing monitoring of inflammatory markers through blood tests.

It's important to note that while managing chronic inflammation is challenging, it is also crucial for long-term health and vitality. By recognizing the triggers and understanding the differences in inflammatory types, you can take proactive steps to safeguard your health against the pervasive effects of chronic inflammation. This might include routine health screenings, adopting a more active lifestyle, and scrutinizing your diet to ensure it supports your body's anti-inflammatory processes.

1.3 Top 10 Common Causes of Inflammation in Everyday Life

In our daily lives, multiple elements contribute to the development of inflammation, often without our conscious awareness. From the foods we eat to the air we breathe, understanding these factors can empower us to make healthier choices. Let's explore some of the most prevalent causes of inflammation that you might encounter regularly.

Dietary Factors

One of the most significant influences on inflammation comes from our diet. Foods high in sugar, trans fats, and excessive alcohol can severely disrupt our body's natural balance. When you consume a lot of sugar, your body experiences a spike in insulin levels, which in turn can trigger an inflammatory response. Foods containing trans fats, often found in processed snacks, baked goods, and some margarines, can raise LDL (bad) cholesterol levels and lower HDL (good) cholesterol levels, contributing to the development of heart disease by fostering inflammatory conditions. Similarly, excessive alcohol consumption can lead to inflammation of the liver (hepatitis), and over time, this can lead to severe liver damage. By understanding these impacts, you can modify your diet to include more anti-inflammatory foods, such as leafy green vegetables, nuts, and fatty fish, which are rich in omega-3 fatty acids.

Environmental Factors

Our environment plays a crucial role in the level of inflammation in our bodies. Pollution, exposure to toxins, and common allergens can all trigger inflammatory responses. For instance, air pollution contains particulate matter that can penetrate deep into the respiratory tract, leading to pulmonary and systemic inflammation. Similarly, exposure to toxic substances like asbestos or high levels of ozone can exacerbate inflammation, particularly in vulnerable populations. Even everyday allergens like pollen, pet dander, or dust mites can provoke our immune systems into an inflammatory response. To mitigate these effects, consider using air purifiers in your home, monitoring air quality indexes in your area before going out, and ensuring your living and working environments are well-ventilated and clean.

Physical Inactivity

In today's world, many of us lead increasingly sedentary lifestyles, which can be detrimental to our health in numerous ways, including increased inflammation. Physical inactivity is associated with the development of obesity and various metabolic diseases, which are themselves inflammatory conditions. Engaging in regular physical activity helps to reduce body fat and the release of inflammatory cytokines associated with adipose tissue. Furthermore, exercise promotes the release of anti-inflammatory substances in the body, helping to counteract any ongoing inflammatory processes. Simple changes, such as incorporating short walks into your daily routine, can significantly impact inflammation levels.

Stress and Sleep

Chronic stress and insufficient sleep are perhaps less obvious but equally significant contributors to inflammation. Stress leads to the release of the hormone cortisol, which, when chronically elevated, can lead to a suppressed immune system and heightened inflammation. Managing stress through techniques such as mindfulness, yoga, or regular physical activity can help maintain healthy cortisol levels. Similarly, poor sleep quality or insufficient sleep can disrupt various body processes, including the regulation of inflammatory responses. Ensuring you get a consistent seven to nine hours of quality sleep per night can significantly reduce inflammation and improve overall health.

By understanding and addressing these common causes of inflammation from your daily environment, diet, activity level, and stress and sleep routines, you can significantly reduce your risk of chronic inflammation and its associated health complications. Making small, manageable changes in these areas can lead to substantial improvements in your overall health and well-being.

1.4 The Connection Between Inflammation and Chronic Diseases

Understanding how chronic inflammation is linked to an array of serious diseases is crucial for anyone looking to maintain optimal health as they age. This persistent, low-grade inflammation acts much like a slow-burning fire within the body, often silently paving the way for long-term health issues such as arthritis, cardiovascular disease, diabetes, and Alzheimer's disease. Each of these conditions has its own unique set of challenges and symptoms, yet the underlying inflammatory processes often share common pathways that can lead to disease progression.

For instance, let's consider arthritis, a group of conditions marked by inflammation in the joints. It's not just the pain and swelling that are problematic but the ongoing nature of the inflammation that can eventually lead to joint damage and loss of mobility. Similarly, in heart disease, chronic inflammation contributes to the buildup of plaque in the arteries, a condition known as atherosclerosis. This plaque buildup is a direct response to injuries caused to the artery walls, which could be due to factors like high blood pressure, smoking, or high cholesterol. Over time, this can lead to heart attacks or strokes as the plaques can rupture, causing clots in the vital arteries of the heart or brain.

Diabetes, particularly type 2, also has a strong inflammatory component. Insulin resistance, a hallmark of type 2 diabetes, involves inflammatory pathways that impair the ability of insulin to work effectively, leading to higher blood sugar levels and, subsequently, various complications such as kidney damage or vision loss. Alzheimer's disease too is increasingly viewed through the lens of inflammation, with researchers finding that chronic inflammation might contribute to the buildup of plaques and tangles in the brain, hallmark features of the disease.

These diseases are not just labels but represent significant alterations in how the body functions, often diminishing the quality of life. Recognizing the role of inflammation in these conditions offers a potential pathway to mitigate risk or possibly slow down the progression through targeted lifestyle and dietary interventions. The presence of certain markers in your blood can signal an elevated inflammatory response. C-reactive protein (CRP) is one such marker, often used by doctors to assess the level of inflammation in the body. Elevated CRP levels are associated with an increased risk of the diseases mentioned, among others. Monitoring these levels can provide crucial insights into your inflammatory status and help guide lifestyle adjustments.

Reflecting on the real-life impacts of these insights, consider the findings from a broad range of studies, including a pivotal 2017 research published in the Journal of Translational Medicine, which showed that reducing inflammation through dietary changes could significantly lower disease risk. This kind of research even this far back underscores the potential power of dietary choices in influencing health outcomes.

In light of these connections, adopting certain lifestyle modifications can be a proactive way to reduce the risk of inflammation-related conditions. Integrating anti-inflammatory foods such as berries, fatty fish, and leafy green vegetables into your diet can make a significant difference. These foods are rich in antioxidants and omega-3 fatty acids, which have been shown to reduce inflammation markers like CRP. Regular physical activity is another powerful tool; even moderate exercise such as walking or swimming can help lower inflammation. Additionally, managing stress through mindfulness practices like yoga or meditation can also reduce the body's inflammatory responses.

The goal here isn't just to add years to your life but to add life to your years by reducing the risk of diseases that can compromise your health and vitality. Making these changes doesn't require drastic overhauls but rather small, manageable shifts in your daily habits that can collectively lead to significant health improvements. By understanding the deep connections between chronic inflammation and disease, and by taking actionable steps towards mitigating these risks, you empower yourself to lead a healthier, more vibrant life.

1.5 How Diet Influences Your Inflammatory Response

The food choices we make each day do more than just satisfy our hunger. They play a critical role in managing the level of inflammation in our bodies. Imagine your diet on a scale, with pro-inflammatory foods on one side and anti-inflammatory foods on the other. Striking the right balance can help tip the scale towards a healthier, less inflamed state. Let's explore how different foods influence inflammation and how you can make choices that help maintain this delicate balance.

Pro-Inflammatory Foods: Certain foods act like fuel for the flames of inflammation. Processed meats, such as sausages and deli meats, contain high levels of advanced glycation end products (AGEs) and saturated fats which can trigger inflammatory processes in the body. Similarly, refined carbohydrates found in white bread, pastries, and other heavily processed foods, rapidly convert to glucose in your bloodstream, spiking blood sugar levels and initiating an inflammatory response. Fried foods, rich in trans fats and unhealthy oils, not only contribute to poor heart health but are also associated with higher levels of inflammation. When consumed in excess, these foods can lead to an imbalance in your body's natural inflammatory response, potentially leading to chronic inflammation and associated diseases.

Anti-Inflammatory Foods: On the flip side, certain foods can help quell inflammation. Foods rich in omega-3 fatty acids, such as salmon, mackerel, and flaxseeds, are renowned for their ability to reduce inflammation. These fats help produce resolvins and protectins, which support ending the inflammatory response in the body. Antioxidants, found abundantly in fruits and vegetables like blueberries, spinach, and bell peppers, help neutralize free radicals that can cause oxidative stress and inflammation. Additionally, dietary fibers found in whole grains, nuts, and legumes help in the production of short-chain fatty acids in the gut, which are potent anti-inflammatory agents.

Consider a day's meals planned with anti-inflammatory foods: start with a breakfast of oatmeal topped with chia seeds and mixed berries, which offer fibers and antioxidants. For lunch, a salad made with mixed greens, cherry tomatoes, and grilled salmon provides a hearty dose of omega-3s and additional antioxidants. A dinner of stir-fried broccoli, carrots, and tofu over quinoa can round out the day with a fiber-rich, nutrient-dense meal that supports your body's anti-inflammatory efforts.

Scientific Evidence: The impact of diet on inflammation is more than just anecdotal; numerous studies back up these claims. Research published in the Journal of the American College of Cardiology highlighted that a diet rich in fruits, vegetables, nuts, whole grains, fish, and unsaturated fat - commonly known as the Mediterranean diet - is associated with lower levels of inflammatory markers like C-reactive protein (CRP) and interleukin-6 (IL-6). Another study from the Harvard School of Public Health found that people who consumed high amounts of sugary beverages and red meat had elevated levels of inflammation, which could be mitigated by dietary changes towards more plant-based, whole-food options.

This solid body of research underscores the profound impact that dietary choices can have on inflammation and, by extension, on our overall health. What you choose to put on your plate can influence your body's inflammatory processes, potentially reducing your risk of chronic diseases and improving your quality of life. As we continue to uncover the complex interactions between diet and health, it becomes increasingly apparent that making informed, mindful food choices is a key component of managing inflammation and supporting long-term health and wellness.

1.6 Debunking Myths: What Inflammation Is and Isn't

In our exploration of inflammation, it's crucial to address some of the most common myths that persist in discussions about this complex biological response. Understanding what inflammation truly entails can empower you to manage your health more effectively and avoid common pitfalls that may hinder your well-being. One widespread misconception is that all inflammation is harmful. This simply isn't the case. As we've discussed, inflammation is a natural and critical process that helps your body heal and defend itself from harm. However, trouble arises when this response becomes chronic, lingering long past the initial threat, potentially leading to various health issues.

Another prevalent myth is that inflammation is always accompanied by pain or visible symptoms. This isn't always true, particularly with chronic inflammation. Often referred to as 'silent inflammation,' it can proceed undetected within your body without obvious symptoms. This type of inflammation is particularly stealthy and dangerous because it can slowly damage your tissues and organs over time, contributing to chronic diseases such as heart disease, diabetes, and Alzheimer's. Understanding that inflammation can be silent is crucial; it underscores the importance of preventive health measures, regular medical check-ups, and being attentive to subtle changes in your body that may indicate underlying issues.

Moving to another important aspect of managing inflammation involves the use of supplements. While anti-inflammatory supplements like turmeric, fish oil, and ginger are popular and can be beneficial, they are not a cure-all solution. The effectiveness of these supplements can vary widely, and they should be used thoughtfully and in conjunction with a healthy diet and lifestyle. For instance, omega-3 supplements can help reduce inflammation and are generally safe for most people. However, high doses may interact with medications or have adverse effects, such as blood thinning. Therefore, it's advisable to consult with a healthcare provider before starting any new supplement regimen, especially if you have existing health conditions or are taking other medications. It is also key to make sure foods and especially any supplementation taken are of high quality as well.

Adopting a holistic approach to managing inflammation is perhaps the most effective strategy. This involves looking at the big picture of your health and considering multiple factors that contribute to inflammation. Diet is a cornerstone of this approach, as certain foods can significantly influence inflammatory processes in your body. Incorporating a variety of anti-inflammatory foods, as discussed previously, can help keep inflammation in check. Physical activity is another crucial element; regular exercise not only helps manage weight and reduce the risk of chronic diseases but also directly contributes to reducing inflammation.

Lifestyle adjustments, such as ensuring adequate sleep and managing stress, are also integral to controlling inflammation. Chronic stress and sleep deprivation can exacerbate inflammatory responses, leading to a cycle that can be hard to break without conscious effort to manage stress and improve sleep quality. Furthermore, medical treatments may also play a role, particularly for individuals dealing with chronic conditions influenced by inflammation. Healthcare professionals can offer guidance on appropriate medications or therapies that can help manage inflammation effectively, tailored to your specific health needs.

In conclusion, understanding the nuances of inflammation and dispelling common myths are essential steps toward taking control of your health. Recognizing that not all inflammation is detrimental, acknowledging that it can occur without noticeable symptoms, using supplements judiciously, and adopting a holistic approach to your lifestyle choices are all strategies that can significantly impact your well-being. By staying informed and proactive, you can navigate the complexities of inflammation and lead a healthier, more vibrant life.

CHAPTER 2
Starting Your Anti-Inflammatory Journey

Imagine standing at a crossroads, one path paved with the foods and habits you've known all your life, and the other leading toward a vibrant, healthier future. Deciding to transition to an anti-inflammatory diet can feel just like that—a pivotal moment that holds the promise of enhanced well-being. It's not merely about reducing inflammation; it's about empowering yourself to make choices that nurture your body and mind. Let this chapter be your guide as you take those initial, decisive steps towards a lifestyle that not only supports your health but also enriches your life.

2.1 First Steps to Transitioning to an Anti-Inflammatory Diet

Initial AssessmentW

Embarking on this transformative path begins with understanding where you stand right now. A food diary is an invaluable tool in this discovery phase. For the next week, I encourage you to write down everything you eat and drink, no matter how small. This record isn't just about capturing your meals; it's about understanding your eating habits, your cravings, and how food integrates into your daily life. Reflect on how you feel after each meal—energized, sluggish, bloated, or satisfied? This introspection can reveal patterns that may be contributing to inflammatory responses in your body, such as a reliance on processed foods, sugars, or trans fats. Recognizing these patterns is the first step in moving toward change.

Goal Setting

With a clearer picture of your current diet, setting realistic goals becomes the next crucial step. Rather than an all-or-nothing approach, aim for balance and gradual integration of anti-inflammatory foods. For instance, set a goal to include a serving of anti-inflammatory foods like berries, nuts, or green leafy vegetables in at least two meals each day. These small, manageable goals are not just easier to stick to; they also accumulate, leading to substantial health benefits over time. Remember, the objective here is progress, not perfection. Each small step you take is a victory worth celebrating.

Introduction to Anti-Inflammatory Food Groups

As you start setting your dietary goals, it's essential to know which foods are your allies in fighting inflammation. Anti-inflammatory foods generally fall into several categories:

- **Omega-3 Rich Foods**: These include fish such as salmon and mackerel, as well as flaxseeds and walnuts. Omega-3 fatty acids are known for their ability to reduce inflammatory markers in the body.

- **Rich in Antioxidants**: Colorful fruits and vegetables like blueberries, oranges, bell peppers, and spinach are packed with antioxidants that combat inflammation by neutralizing free radicals in the body.

- **Whole Grains and Fiber**: Foods like oatmeal, brown rice, and whole wheat help reduce inflammation by maintaining healthy digestion and promoting the growth of beneficial gut bacteria.

- **Herbs and Spices**: Turmeric, ginger, garlic, and cinnamon are not just flavorful—they also contain powerful compounds that reduce inflammation.

Incorporating a variety of these foods into your diet can significantly reduce inflammation and support overall health.

Gradual Integration

For many, the idea of overhauling their diet overnight is daunting and unsustainable. Instead, I advocate for a gradual approach to dietary changes. Start by introducing one new anti-inflammatory food into your diet each week. For example, you might add a handful of nuts to your breakfast routine or swap your usual snack for a piece of fresh fruit. As these foods become staples in your diet, you'll likely notice subtle improvements in how you feel each day. This method not only eases the transition but also helps build lasting habits by allowing you to experience and adapt to changes at your own pace.

Navigating the shift to an anti-inflammatory diet is not about rigid dietary restrictions or perfection; it's about making smarter choices that enhance your health. Each positive change is a step towards a more vibrant version of yourself, fueled not just by the foods you eat but by a deeper understanding of how these foods affect your body. As you continue on this path, remember that every meal is an opportunity to nourish your body and invest in your long-term well-being.

2.2 Setting Up Your Kitchen for Success: Essential Tools and Ingredients

Creating an environment that supports your new eating habits is just as crucial as the food choices you make. Think of your kitchen as the heart of your home where good health begins. Equipping it with the right tools and organizing it for efficiency can transform the way you cook and influence your nutritional habits. Let's explore how setting up your kitchen can make preparing anti-inflammatory meals not only easier but also more enjoyable.

Kitchen Tools

A well-stocked kitchen is your best ally in preparing meals that are both delicious and health-supportive. Start with a good set of sharp knives. A chef's knife and a paring knife can handle most of your chopping and slicing needs, making meal prep quicker and safer. Consider investing in a high-quality blender as well; it's indispensable for making smoothies, soups, and purees rich in fruits and vegetables. A large cutting board, several mixing bowls of various sizes, and a set of measuring cups and spoons are also essential. These tools will help you handle fresh produce and whole ingredients more efficiently, encouraging you to use them more often. Additionally, a spice grinder can be a fantastic tool, allowing you to use whole spices, which retain their flavor and potent anti-inflammatory properties longer than their pre-ground counterparts.

Pantry Staples

Stocking your pantry with a selection of anti-inflammatory staples is like having a treasure trove at your fingertips, ready to enhance any meal. Spices such as turmeric and ginger are not only flavorful but are also renowned for their anti-inflammatory properties; incorporating these into your diet can boost your health significantly. Keep a variety of whole grains like quinoa, oats, and brown rice on hand. These are excellent sources of fiber, which helps control blood sugar levels and supports digestive health. Legumes, including beans, lentils, and chickpeas, are also essential. They're versatile, nutritious, and a great plant-based protein source, making them perfect for numerous dishes from salads to soups. Nuts and seeds, such as almonds, chia seeds, and flaxseeds, are great for snacks and add crunch and nutrients to dishes. These staples not only enrich your diet but also ensure that you have the necessary ingredients to prepare anti-inflammatory meals whenever you need them.

Storage Tips

Proper storage of your food preserves its nutritional value and flavor, making your cooking both healthier and more tasty. Store spices in a cool, dark place to maintain their essential oils and flavors—these are the components that contribute to their anti-inflammatory effects. Nuts and seeds can go rancid quickly due to their high-fat content, so keep them in airtight containers in the refrigerator or freezer. This keeps them fresh and preserves their beneficial fats, which are crucial for reducing inflammation. For whole grains and legumes, opt for clear, airtight containers that not only keep them fresh but also let you see what you have at a glance, reducing waste and making meal planning easier.

Organizational Tips

The way you organize your kitchen can significantly impact the ease with which you prepare your meals. Place fruits and vegetables on the middle shelf of your refrigerator or in a produce drawer at eye level. When healthy choices are the first thing you see, you're more likely to choose them over less healthy options. Organize your pantry in zones; designate specific areas for spices, another for whole grains, and another for canned goods. This not only saves you time when cooking but also helps you keep track of your inventory, which is crucial for maintaining a well-stocked kitchen. Consider using turntables in your cabinets for spices and condiments; this makes it easier to find what you need without having to dig through a cluttered space.

Setting up your kitchen with these tools and systems transforms it into a space that supports your anti-inflammatory diet. It makes healthy cooking practical and enjoyable, encouraging you to stick with your dietary changes in the long term. As you continue to adapt your eating habits, remember that the layout of your kitchen and the tools you use can be just as important as the food you choose to eat. This supportive environment not only makes it easier to prepare nourishing meals but also turns cooking into a pleasure, helping you to embrace and maintain your new healthy lifestyle with ease.

2.3 Understanding Food Labels and Inflammatory Additives to Avoid

Navigating the aisles of your local grocery store is more than a shopping trip; it's a tour through a minefield of potential inflammatory triggers hidden in plain sight on food labels. Learning to decipher these labels is akin to learning a new language—one that can significantly impact your health and wellness. When you pick up a product and turn it over to read the ingredients, you're taking an important step toward making informed choices about what you put into your body. Let's delve into how you can become fluent in the language of food labels, highlighting inflammatory ingredients to avoid and healthier alternatives to embrace.

The first step in mastering food label literacy is understanding that not all ingredients are created equal. Focus on identifying added sugars and trans fats, which are notorious for their inflammatory effects. Added sugars can appear under various names—anything ending in 'ose', such as fructose or sucrose, is a clue, as well as terms like cane sugar, corn syrup, or maltose. These sugars, when consumed in excess, can kickstart inflammatory processes in your body, leading to chronic inflammation over time. Trans fats, often listed as 'partially hydrogenated oils', are equally detrimental. Found in many baked goods, snacks, and fried foods, trans fats contribute to inflammation and are linked to an increased risk of heart disease.

Another category to watch out for includes certain preservatives and additives that can induce inflammation. Monosodium glutamate (MSG), often used to enhance flavor in processed foods, can lead to inflammation and adverse reactions in some individuals. Similarly, high-fructose corn syrup, a common sweetener in sodas and sweetened beverages, is not only a source of excessive sugar but also a catalyst for inflammation. By identifying these ingredients on labels, you can make choices that align better with your anti-inflammatory objectives.

Switching to healthier alternatives is about making simple substitutions without compromising on taste or satisfaction. Instead of products laden with added sugars, look for those sweetened naturally with fruits, honey, or even pure maple syrup—these offer sweetness along with nutritional benefits. For healthy fats, opt for natural sources like avocado oil or extra virgin olive oil instead of items containing trans fats. These natural oils provide beneficial fats that can help to reduce inflammation in the body.

Understanding food certifications and claims can also guide you in making better choices. Products labeled 'organic' ensure that the ingredients have been grown without synthetic pesticides and fertilizers, which can contribute to inflammation. Similarly, items certified 'non-GMO' are free from genetically modified organisms, which some choose to avoid to reduce exposure to potential inflammatory agents. While these labels aren't a direct indicator of anti-inflammatory properties, they often point to higher-quality ingredients that align better with a health-conscious diet.

Becoming proficient in reading food labels and understanding what they tell you about the contents is a powerful tool in your anti-inflammatory diet. It allows you to avoid hidden triggers and choose ingredients that support rather than challenge your health. Each time you choose to avoid a harmful ingredient, you're taking a positive step towards better health and reduced inflammation. Remember, every product you put back on the shelf is a testament to your commitment to your wellness.

2.4 Simple Swaps: Replacing Common Inflammatory Foods

Adopting an anti-inflammatory diet doesn't necessarily mean a complete overhaul of your eating habits. Often, it's about making smarter choices by swapping out foods that trigger inflammation for healthier alternatives. This approach not only eases the transition but also supports sustainable change. Let's explore some simple substitutions that can significantly reduce your dietary inflammation.

Dairy Alternatives

For many individuals, dairy products can be a primary source of inflammation, often due to lactose intolerance or a sensitivity to the proteins found in cow's milk. Symptoms like bloating, gas, and digestive discomfort after consuming dairy are tell-tale signs that your body might not be responding well to these products. Replacing traditional milk with plant-based alternatives can offer relief and contribute to reducing inflammation. Almond milk, for instance, is a popular choice that's not only low in calories but also free of the lactose and proteins that can trigger inflammatory responses. It's a versatile substitute that works well in everything from your morning cereal to coffee and smoothies. Coconut milk is another excellent alternative, especially for cooking, as it adds a creamy texture aWnd a hint of sweetness to dishes without the inflammatory effects of dairy. For those who enjoy yogurt, coconut yogurt can be a delightful alternative, offering the same probiotic benefits without the potential drawbacks of dairy. These substitutions not only help manage inflammation but also diversify your diet with new flavors and textures.

Healthy Fats

As we touched on above, the fats you choose to consume can have a significant impact on your inflammation levels. Many processed foods contain unhealthy fats such as trans fats or excessive saturated fats, found in products like margarine, which can exacerbate inflammation. Swapping these out for healthier fats can markedly improve your health. Avocado oil and extra virgin olive oil are excellent choices. Avocado oil is not only high in monounsaturated fats, which are good for heart health, but it also has a high smoke point, making it ideal for cooking at higher temperatures without breaking down into harmful compounds. Extra virgin olive oil, a staple of the anti-inflammatory Mediterranean diet, is rich in polyphenols, antioxidants that have been shown to reduce inflammation. Integrating these oils into your cooking can significantly reduce the inflammatory impact of your meals. Use them for sautéing vegetables or as a base for dressings and sauces to enrich your dishes with both flavor and nutritional benefits.

Sweetener Solutions

You know I couldn't write a book without talking about SUG-

AR! Reducing your intake of refined sugars is crucial in managing inflammation. High consumption of refined sugars triggers a cascade of inflammatory responses that can lead to increased levels of chronic inflammation. Natural sweeteners like honey and stevia offer a solution. Honey, while still sweet, contains antioxidants and nutrients that refined sugars lack, providing some defensive benefits against inflammation. It also has antimicrobial properties, which can support your overall health. Stevia, a natural sweetener derived from the leaves of the Stevia plant, contains no calories and does not increase blood sugar levels, making it an excellent option for those managing diabetes or looking to reduce calorie intake. Incorporating these natural sweeteners into your diet instead of sugar can help mitigate the inflammatory response typically associated with high sugar intake. I love my sweets as much as anyone, so I understand this can be a challenge. Once you get a few good days under your belt, your body will feel better and that is SO motivating to keep going!

Snack Replacements

Snacking can be a significant source of inflammatory foods due to the prevalence of processed options that are high in sugar, unhealthy fats, and artificial additives-the trifecta. Replacing these snacks with healthier alternatives is a straightforward way to reduce inflammation. Instead of reaching for a bag of store-bought potato chips, try making your own kale chips. Kale is high in vitamins and antioxidants, which help combat inflammation. Simply toss chopped kale leaves in a little olive oil, sprinkle with a pinch of salt, and bake them in the oven until crisp. Not only are these homemade chips delicious and satisfying, but they also provide a nutrient boost without the inflammatory effects of commercially fried snacks. This swap not only enhances your nutrient intake but also reduces your consumption of the unhealthy oils and additives found in many snack foods.

Each of these simple swaps represents a step toward a healthier, more balanced diet that supports reducing inflammation. By choosing plant-based dairy alternatives, healthier fats, natural sweeteners, and nutritious snacks, you're not only mitigating inflammatory responses but also enhancing your overall dietary quality. These changes, while simple, can have profound effects on your health and well-being, helping you feel better each day as you continue to make choices that support your body's needs.

2.5 The Importance of a Slow and Steady Approach

Change, especially when it relates to lifestyle and diet, is easier to handle mentally when approached gradually. Embracing this concept is crucial as you adapt to an anti-inflammatory diet. Quick fixes might offer immediate satisfaction, but they rarely lead to lasting health benefits. Instead, integrating slow and steady changes into your lifestyle allows you to build habits that are sustainable in the long term. This method is supported by behavioral science, which suggests that gradual changes help to rewire our habits in ways that are more likely to stick. When you make a small change, like swapping a daily soda for a glass of water, you begin to form new neural pathways in your brain that reinforce this healthier choice. Over time, these small changes accumulate and become your new norm, making it easier to maintain these healthier habits without feeling overwhelmed or deprived.

Setting achievable milestones is another key aspect of this approach. Instead of aiming to overhaul your diet in one go, set smaller, more manageable goals that lead to big results over time. For instance, you might start by introducing one anti-inflammatory food into each meal or cooking a healthy meal at home three times a week. These goals should feel achievable and tailored to your current lifestyle, which helps prevent the discouragement that often comes with more ambitious goals. Celebrating these small victories can also boost your motivation to continue. Each healthy choice is a step forward, and recognizing your progress is essential for maintaining morale and commitment. I like to have mini rewards for myself that are not food-related. When I make a healthy habit change and stick to it for, say, one month, then I will get a manicure or go to a movie. Something non-food that celebrates my accomplishment. More on this later in Chapter 6.

Regularly monitoring your progress is vital for understanding the impact of your dietary changes. This can be as simple as keeping a journal where you note your meals, how you feel, and any new symptoms or improvements in your health. Alternatively, numerous apps can help track your eating habits, symptoms, and even provide insights into nutrient intake. This regular monitoring not only helps you stay on track but also allows you to see the tangible benefits of your dietary changes. For instance, you might notice an improvement in your energy levels or a reduction in digestive discomfort. These positive changes serve as powerful motivation to continue with your anti-inflammatory diet.

Patience is your greatest ally in this process. Changing dietary habits is a journey that requires time and adjustment. It's natural to encounter setbacks or days when you don't meet your goals. What's important is how you respond to these challenges. Instead of viewing them as failures, see them as opportunities to learn and adapt your approach. Maybe a particular goal was too ambitious, or life got in the way—adjust your plans accordingly and continue forward. It's also crucial to listen to your body and be willing to make adjustments based on your responses. Everyone's body is different, and what works for one person may not work for another. Being open to tweaking your diet in response to how you feel can help you find the balance that works best for you. Show yourself grace.

By embracing a slow and steady approach, setting achievable milestones, monitoring your progress, and practicing patience, you create a foundation for lasting health improvements. This method not only makes the transition to an anti-inflammatory diet more manageable but also increases the likelihood that these healthier habits will become a permanent part of your lifestyle. As you continue to make these gradual changes, remember that each step forward is a positive move towards a healthier, more vibrant you.

2.6 How to Read Your Body's Responses to Diet Changes

As you adapt to an anti-inflammatory diet, your body begins a remarkable process of adjustment and healing, which can manifest in various ways. Recognizing and understanding these signals can significantly enhance your ability to sustain these dietary changes and truly reap the benefits. When you start feeding your body the right mix of nutrients and reduce your intake of inflammatory foods, you'll notice several positive changes. One of the first signs many people experience is a reduction in bloating. This decrease in abdominal discomfort and swelling is often the result of cutting out foods that your body may struggle to digest or that trigger inflammatory responses. Who doesn't love a flatter belly?? Another encouraging sign is an increase in energy levels. It's like rediscovering a zest for life that you didn't realize was missing. You might find yourself feeling more active, willing to engage in physical activities, or simply feeling less sluggish throughout the day. No more 3 pm nap (or coffee) needed.

Clearer skin is another visible benefit that often delights those who switch to an anti-inflammatory diet. This can be particularly evident if your diet previously included a lot of sugar, dairy, or processed foods, which can exacerbate skin issues like acne or eczema. As your diet improves, your skin often reflects these changes, becoming clearer and more vibrant. The skin is the largest detoxing organ. Each of these changes is a clear signal from your body that the dietary choices you're making are beneficial and that your internal environment is becoming less inflamed and more balanced.

However, it's not uncommon to experience some detox symptoms as you transition away from inflammatory foods. These symptoms can include headaches, fatigue, or even a temporary increase in joint discomfort. These are natural reactions as your body begins to expel toxins and adjust to the absence of its usual sugar and fat overloads. While these symptoms can be uncomfortable, they are usually short-lived and should subside as your body adapts to the healthier dietary regimen. It's important during this phase to stay well-hydrated and get plenty of rest to support your body's adjustment process.

Over the longer term, there are key health markers you should monitor to gauge the impact of your new eating habits. Two of the most significant are your cholesterol levels and blood pressure, both of which can see marked improvement on an anti-inflammatory diet. Lowering the intake of unhealthy fats and increasing your consumption of whole grains, fruits, and vegetables can help reduce "bad" LDL cholesterol and improve "good" HDL cholesterol levels. Similarly, reducing salt intake and increasing potassium-rich foods can help lower blood pressure. Monitoring these markers can not only motivate you by showing tangible benefits but also help you tweak your diet to target these areas specifically.

Embracing an anti-inflammatory diet is about tuning in to your body and listening to the signals it sends. By paying attention to both the positive changes and the signs of detoxing, and by keeping an eye on crucial health markers, you can navigate your way through this transition with confidence.

Reflecting on the Journey

As we close this chapter, it's vital to acknowledge the transformation your body undergoes as you embrace an anti-inflammatory lifestyle. The signs of positive change, understanding detoxing symptoms, and monitoring long-term health markers are all crucial elements that guide you through this adaptation. Each step you take builds upon the last, creating a healthier version of yourself not just for today, but for many years to come.

In the next chapter, we will explore how to maintain these dietary changes amidst the complexities of modern life, ensuring that you can sustain this healthier way of living regardless of the challenges you may face.

CHAPTER 3
Anti-Inflammatory Recipes for Beginners

Imagine waking up each morning feeling refreshed, energized, and ready to embrace the day. What if I told you that such mornings are not just a dream, but could be your new reality? The secret lies in beginning your day with meals that not only tantalize your taste buds but also help combat inflammation, setting a positive tone for your day. This chapter is your guide to transforming your mornings with delicious, anti-inflammatory breakfasts that are simple to prepare and packed with benefits that extend well beyond your morning routine.

3.1 5 Quick Breakfasts to Start an Anti-Inflammatory Day

Smoothie Solutions

Starting your day with a smoothie is an excellent way to infuse your body with nutrients while keeping inflammation at bay. Smoothies are incredibly versatile, and by incorporating ingredients such as spinach, avocado, berries, and flaxseed, you create a powerhouse beverage that supports your health from the first sip. Here's a simple recipe to get you started: blend one cup of spinach, half an avocado, a cup of mixed berries (blueberries, strawberries, and raspberries work wonderfully), a tablespoon of ground flaxseed, and a cup of almond milk. This blend not only offers a rich array of antioxidants from the berries and spinach but also includes healthy fats from the avocado and flaxseed, which are excellent for managing inflammation. What's more, it's ready in minutes, making it perfect for those busy mornings when time is of the essence.

Overnight Oats Variants

Overnight oats are a fantastic option for anyone looking to prepare their breakfasts ahead of time. The beauty of overnight oats lies in their simplicity and the endless variations you can create to keep your mornings interesting. To start, mix half a cup of rolled oats with one cup of your preferred milk or yogurt, a tablespoon of chia seeds, and a sprinkle of cinnamon in a jar. Let this mixture soak overnight in the refrigerator. In the morning, top it with a handful of almonds for crunch and a drizzle of honey for a touch of sweetness. This breakfast is not only filling but also packed with ingredients like chia seeds and cinnamon, which possess natural anti-inflammatory properties, helping you to start your day on a healthy note.

Egg Dishes Redefined

Eggs are a breakfast staple and for a good reason. They're versatile, protein-rich, and when prepared with anti-inflammatory ingredients, can be an excellent start to your day. Try scrambling your eggs with a dash of turmeric, a powerful anti-inflammatory spice that gives your meal a vibrant color and a healthful boost. Add some diced bell peppers, spinach, and onions for a vegetable-packed meal that's both nutritious and satisfying. Alternatively, for those who enjoy a heartier breakfast, a vegetable omelet with fresh herbs like parsley and chives can be a delightful option. These dishes are not just delicious; they're also a great way to incorporate a variety of anti-inflammatory foods into your morning routine. A whole muffin pan of these can be made once a week and stored in the fridge. Then just heat and eat!

Gluten-Free Pancakes

For those who love a sweet start to the day, pancakes can be a comforting choice. Making them anti-inflammatory and gluten-free is easier than you might think. Start with a base of almond flour, which is not only gluten-free but also contains magnesium, a mineral known for its anti-inflammatory properties. Mix one cup of almond flour, one teaspoon of baking powder, a pinch of salt, two eggs, a quarter cup of almond milk, and a tablespoon of honey. Cook them as you would traditional pancakes and serve them topped with a mix of anti-inflammatory berries like blueberries and raspberries and a drizzle of honey. This dish proves that you can enjoy a sweet breakfast without the inflammatory effects of refined sugars and gluten.

Each of these breakfast options is designed to provide a balanced, nutrient-rich start to your day, with a focus on ease and flavor. By incorporating these meals into your morning routine, you not only nourish your body but also take an important step towards reducing inflammation and enhancing your overall well-being. Enjoy the blend of flavors and the health benefits they bring, knowing that each bite is a step towards a healthier you.

3.2 Lunches on the Go: Simple and Quick Anti-Inflammatory Options

When midday hunger strikes, especially during a busy day, having a nutritious, anti-inflammatory meal ready can make all the difference in maintaining your energy and health. These lunch options are designed to be easy to prepare, delicious to enjoy, and portable enough to take with you, whether it's to the office or a kid's sporting weekend.

Wraps and rolls offer a versatile and delightful way to enjoy a variety of anti-inflammatory ingredients. Imagine a wrap made with a large, fresh collard green leaf, sturdy enough to hold a generous filling yet tender enough to bite through easily. Inside this green envelope, you could layer grilled chicken breast, sliced and seasoned with a pinch of black pepper and a squeeze of fresh lemon juice for zest. Add slices of creamy avocado, rich in monounsaturated fats known to help reduce inflammation, and a rainbow of vegetables such as shredded purple cabbage, carrot matchsticks, and thinly sliced cucumbers for crunch and color. Roll it tightly, and you have a handheld meal that is not only satisfying but also packed with nutrients that fight inflammation. For those who prefer grains, a whole-grain tortilla can substitute for the collard green, adding a comforting, hearty base to the wrap.

Salads are a lunchtime staple, and a 'salad in a jar' is a creative twist that enhances both the visual appeal and the practicality of this dish. Start with a homemade dressing at the base—perhaps a vibrant ginger and turmeric vinaigrette, both known for their anti-inflammatory properties. Pour this into a jar, and then begin layering your ingredients, starting with the heaviest and most non-absorbent at the bottom to keep them from becoming soggy. Add a layer of chickpeas or cooked quinoa for protein, followed by a variety of colorful vegetables. Think cherry tomatoes, sliced bell peppers, and a handful of baby spinach. Top the jar with seeds or nuts for a crunch—pumpkin seeds or slivered almonds work beautifully. When you're ready to eat, just shake the jar to distribute the dressing through the salad. This not only mixes the flavors beautifully but also keeps your meal fresh until you're ready to enjoy it.

Quinoa salad is another excellent choice for a nutritious, anti-inflammatory lunch. Quinoa, a seed rather than a grain, provides a complete protein source, which is rare in plant foods and fantastic for your health. For a simple yet delicious quinoa salad, mix cooked quinoa with black beans, cherry tomatoes, and cucumbers—all ingredients noted for their fiber content and anti-inflammatory properties. Add a dressing made from lime juice, olive oil, and a hint of cumin for an extra kick. This salad can be made in large batches and stored in the fridge, making it a perfect option for meal prep days when you plan your meals for the week.

Lastly, soups are a comforting and convenient lunch option, especially when you need something warm during cooler days. A ginger carrot soup, for example, can be a fantastic anti-inflammatory choice. Ginger offers potent anti-inflammatory benefits, and carrots are high in beta-carotene, which your body converts into vitamin A, known for its immune-boosting properties. To make the soup, sauté onions and garlic in olive oil until soft, add chopped carrots and grated fresh ginger, then pour in vegetable broth and let simmer until the carrots are tender. Blend the mixture until smooth for a creamy finish. This soup can be made ahead of time and carried in a thermos for a warm, satisfying midday meal.

These lunch options are designed not just to satisfy your hunger but to soothe inflammation and boost your overall health. They are simple to prepare, easy to customize with your favorite ingredients, and perfect for taking on the go, ensuring that even on your busiest days, you can nourish your body with what it needs to thrive.

3.3 Stress-Free Dinners: One-Pot Anti-Inflammatory Meals

When evening rolls around, the last thing you want is to be tied up in the kitchen for hours. Instead, imagine serving a dinner that not only bursts with flavor and color but also supports your health with every bite. One-pot meals are the answer to this dream. They simplify cooking and cleaning, allowing more time for you to relax and enjoy the company of loved ones. Let's explore some delightful one-pot recipes that are as easy on your time as they are on your body's inflammatory responses.

Stir-Fry Techniques

A vibrant vegetable stir-fry can turn your dinner into a festive yet healthful feast. Begin with a base of aromatic ingredients like minced garlic and grated ginger sautéed in a splash of sesame oil. These flavors not only set the stage for a delicious meal but also pack a punch in terms of health benefits, especially ginger with its potent anti-inflammatory properties. Once these aromatics are golden and fragrant, elevate your stir-fry by adding a rainbow of vegetables. Think bright bell peppers, crisp snap peas, and tender broccoli florets. For protein, tofu cubes or shrimp are excellent choices; they're not only quick to cook but also align well with the anti-inflammatory theme. Tofu, in particular, is a great plant-based protein that beautifully absorbs the flavors of your stir-fry sauce—a simple mix of low-sodium soy sauce, a touch of honey, and a splash of rice vinegar. This dish cooks in minutes, and the variety of vegetables provides a spectrum of antioxidants and nutrients, making your dinner both a health booster and a visual delight.

One-Pot Vegan Curries

There's something incredibly comforting about a bowl of curry. Its warmth and complexity of flavors make it a beloved dish for many. For a healthful twist, a vegan curry that utilizes the anti-inflammatory powers of spices like turmeric, cumin, and coriander is perfect. Start by sautéing onions, garlic, and a knob of fresh ginger in coconut oil until they're soft and starting to brown. Add your ground spices, stirring until the kitchen fills with their warm aromas. Pour in a can of coconut milk for creaminess and add a variety of chopped vegetables like carrots, bell peppers, and zucchini. Chickpeas or lentils can also be tossed into the mix for protein. Let the curry simmer until the vegetables are tender. Each spoonful of this curry isn't just delicious; it's packed with spices known for their anti-inflammatory effects, making it a powerful ally for your health.

Slow Cooker Successes

The slow cooker is a marvelous tool for anyone looking to reduce kitchen time without sacrificing the quality and health benefits of their meals. A slow-cooked chicken stew with sweet potatoes and kale is a case in point. Start by placing diced sweet potatoes and carrots at the bottom of the slow cooker, adding a layer of seasoned chicken thighs on top, and then covering everything with chicken broth. About an hour before serving, stir in some roughly chopped kale, allowing it to wilt and absorb the flavors of the stew. The slow cooking process enhances the flavors and textures of the ingredients while preserving their nutritional content. Sweet potatoes are also high in beta-carotene while kale adds a wealth of vitamins and minerals. Set your slow cooker in the morning and come home to a delectable, ready-to-eat dinner that supports your anti-inflammatory diet with minimal effort.

Sheet Pan Meals

For those who value simplicity and minimal cleanup, sheet pan meals are a fantastic solution. A favorite combination might include placing fillets of salmon alongside halves of Brussels sprouts and cubed sweet potatoes on a single sheet pan. Drizzle everything with a mix of olive oil, lemon juice, and a sprinkle of herbs like dill or rosemary, which not only add flavor but also possess their own anti-inflammatory benefits. Roast in a preheated oven until the salmon is flaky and vegetables are tender and caramelized. This meal requires minimal preparation and cleanup, yet delivers maximum flavor and nutritional benefits. The omega-3 fatty acids in salmon are excellent for reducing inflammation, while Brussels sprouts and sweet potatoes provide fiber, antioxidants, and other vital nutrients to support overall health.

Each of these dinner options highlights how easy it can be to incorporate anti-inflammatory eating into even the busiest of schedules. These meals prove that you don't need to spend hours in the kitchen to enjoy a healthful, delicious dinner that supports your well-being. Whether you're stirring, simmering, slow-cooking, or roasting, these recipes offer stress-free paths to a satisfying end to your day.

3.4 Snacks and Sides: Easy, Tasty, and Inflammation-Free

When mid-afternoon hunger pangs strike, reaching for the right snack can make all the difference in how you feel for the rest of the day. Instead of settling for processed options that might aggravate inflammation, why not indulge in homemade snacks that are not only delicious but also help soothe and reduce inflammation? Homemade veggie chips, for instance, are a wonderful alternative to store-bought snacks, which often come loaded with unhealthy oils and preservatives. Making your own chips at home, such as sweet potato chips, allows you to control the ingredients and incorporate anti-inflammatory spices like turmeric or rosemary for an added health boost. For sweet potato chips, thin slice, season, and spread them on a baking sheet and bake at a low temperature until crispy. These chips not only satisfy your crunchy cravings but also provide valuable nutrients bolstering your diet with anti-inflammatory benefits.

Dips and spreads are another fantastic snack option, and homemade hummus is a standout choice. Rich in protein and fiber, hummus is made primarily from chickpeas, tahini, lemon juice, and garlic—all ingredients known for their health benefits. By adding roasted garlic or red peppers, you not only enhance the flavor profile but also pack in antioxidants that help fight inflammation. Roasted red pepper hummus, for example, can be made by blending cooked chickpeas with tahini, a roasted red pepper, a clove of roasted garlic, a squeeze of lemon, and a dash of cumin. The result is a creamy, flavorful spread that goes wonderfully with raw vegetables or whole-grain crackers, providing a satisfying snack that supports your anti-inflammatory diet.

Nuts and seeds are invaluable in an anti-inflammatory diet, offering a potent combination of proteins, healthy fats, and various micronutrients that help manage inflammation. Creating your own nut and seed mix gives you the freedom to choose your favorite varieties and add spices that further enhance their anti-inflammatory properties. A mix of walnuts, almonds, and pumpkin seeds, lightly toasted and sprinkled with a pinch of sea salt and turmeric, can be a fantastic snack option. Walnuts are rich in omega-3 fatty acids, almonds provide a good dose of vitamin E, and pumpkin seeds are a great source of magnesium—all nutrients that play a role in reducing inflammation. This mix not only packs a nutritional punch but also keeps you full and satisfied between meals, making it easier to resist less healthful snacks.

For a sweet treat that doesn't sacrifice your health goals, fruit-based snacks are a delightful solution. Simple yet delicious, an apple sliced and spread with a thin layer of almond butter offers a satisfying crunch with a hint of creaminess. The apple provides fiber and vitamin C, while almond butter adds protein and healthy fats, making this snack both nutritious and comforting. Alternatively, a berry and yogurt parfait can serve as a refreshing and healthful snack or dessert. Layer Greek yogurt with a mixture of fresh berries and a sprinkle of flaxseeds for a snack that's rich in antioxidants, protein, and omega-3 fatty acids. Not only are these fruit-based snacks incredibly tasty, but they also support your body's anti-inflammatory processes, helping you feel revitalized and nourished.

Each of these snack options is designed to be easy to prepare, delicious to eat, and beneficial for your health, aligning perfectly with an anti-inflammatory lifestyle. By choosing to make these snacks at home, you not only enjoy fresher, tastier results but also gain the peace of mind that comes from knowing exactly what you're eating. Whether you crave something savory like veggie chips and hummus or something sweet like fruit and yogurt, these snacks ensure you're nourished, satisfied, and on track with your health goals. Make snack time a key part of your daily wellness routine.

3.5 Sweet Treats: Anti-Inflammatory Desserts That Delight

Indulging in a sweet treat doesn't have to mean straying from your anti-inflammatory diet. In fact, with a few clever substitutions and the right ingredients, you can prepare desserts that not only satisfy your sweet tooth but also contribute to your health. These dessert recipes are crafted to delight your senses while infusing your body with anti-inflammatory benefits. Let's explore how desserts can be both a luxurious treat and a healthful part of your day.

Fruit Sorbets

One of the simplest pleasures on a warm day, or really any day, is a refreshing sorbet. Made with ripe, anti-inflammatory fruits like mangoes and pineapples, these sorbets are naturally sweet, incredibly refreshing, and brimming with health benefits. To create a mango sorbet, start by pureeing fresh or frozen mango chunks until smooth. Enhance the natural sweetness with a touch of honey or agave nectar, both of which are more favorable alternatives to refined sugar. For a bit of complexity and a boost in anti-inflammatory power, add a squeeze of fresh lime juice and a pinch of grated ginger. Freeze the mixture until solid, then pulse briefly in a food processor to achieve a silky texture before serving. Pineapple sorbet can be made similarly, capitalizing on pineapple's bromelain content, an enzyme known for its anti-inflammatory and digestive benefits. These sorbets are not just a treat for your palate but also a soothing remedy for your body, providing hydration and nutrients while cooling you down.

Dark Chocolate Treats

Dark chocolate, especially varieties containing 70% cocoa or more, is a well-known anti-inflammatory food, thanks to its high levels of flavonoids. These compounds help reduce inflammation and increase blood flow, making dark chocolate not just a permissible indulgence but a beneficial one. For a simple yet elegant dessert, try dark chocolate-dipped strawberries. Melt dark chocolate over a double boiler, then dip fresh strawberries into the chocolate, letting the excess drip off before setting them on a parchment-lined tray. Chill in the refrigerator until the chocolate sets. The sweetness of the strawberries complements the bitterness of the dark chocolate, creating a sophisticated flavor profile. Similarly, dark chocolate-dipped almonds offer a satisfying crunch and are a great way to get a dose of healthy fats, protein, and the antioxidant benefits of dark chocolate in a portable, convenient form. These also make a great sweet gift! Imagine if we all swapped healthy treats rather than heavy cookies or processed foods that actually make us feel bad. Give the gift of health.

Baked Fruit Dishes

Baked fruit dishes are a wonderful way to enjoy the natural sweetness of fruits while enhancing their flavor with warm, comforting spices that also boast anti-inflammatory properties. Cinnamon-baked apples are a classic dish that is simple to prepare and so comforting. Core a few apples and place them in a baking dish. Mix a filling of rolled oats, chopped nuts, a sprinkle of cinnamon, and a drizzle of honey, then stuff the apples with this mixture. Bake until the apples are tender and the filling is golden. Another delightful option is roasted pears. Halve and core some pears, placing them cut-side up in a baking dish. Drizzle with a little honey and sprinkle with cinnamon and nutmeg before baking until just softened. These dishes transform the humble fruits into warm, soothing desserts that not only satisfy your dessert cravings but also provide the benefits of fiber, vitamins, and anti-inflammatory spices.

Avocado Chocolate Mousse

Avocado chocolate mousse is a dessert that truly embodies the idea of indulgence without guilt. Avocados provide a creamy base rich in healthy fats, fiber, and a variety of essential nutrients, all of which contribute to reducing inflammation. To make this mousse, blend ripe avocados with high-quality cocoa powder, a touch of maple syrup for sweetness, and a splash of vanilla extract for depth of flavor. The result is a rich, creamy mousse that rivals any traditional chocolate dessert in both texture and taste, yet much better supports your health. Serve chilled with a sprinkle of shaved dark chocolate or a few raspberries for an added antioxidant boost.

These dessert recipes show that a focus on anti-inflammatory ingredients doesn't mean sacrificing flavor or enjoyment. Each recipe offers a delicious way to end a meal or treat yourself during the day, providing not just pleasure but also a wealth of health benefits. Enjoy these sweet treats knowing they are crafted to delight both your taste buds and support your well-being.

3.6 Weekend Specials: Family Meals to Share and Enjoy

Creating meals that bring the family together around the dining table is one of the joys of home cooking. When these meals are also designed to reduce inflammation, they bring an additional layer of care and health benefits to your loved ones. This section offers a variety of recipes that are perfect for leisurely weekend cooking, focusing on dishes that are both delightful to share and beneficial for health.

Family-Style Roasts

Roasting is a culinary technique that not only enhances the flavor of meats and vegetables but also preserves their nutrients, making them healthier. For a family-style meal that is as nourishing as it is satisfying, consider preparing an herb-roasted chicken or leg of lamb. Begin with a free-range chicken or a piece of grass-fed lamb, as these are higher in anti-inflammatory omega-3 fatty acids compared to their conventionally raised counterparts. Generously rub the meat with a mix of chopped herbs such as rosemary, thyme, and oregano, all known for their anti-inflammatory properties, along with a dash of olive oil and garlic. Surround the meat with a variety of vegetables like carrots, sweet potatoes, and onions. These not only cook alongside the main protein, absorbing the rich flavors, but they also bring their own set of anti-inflammatory benefits, notably from the beta-carotene in the carrots and the quercetin in the onions. Roast until the meat is tender and the vegetables are caramelized. This meal not only fills the house with enticing aromas but also provides a hearty, healthful meal that everyone can enjoy.

Fish Tacos with Coleslaw

Fish tacos are a fun and informal way to gather the family, allowing everyone to customize their plate. Start with a good-quality white fish, such as cod or tilapia, known for their lean protein and omega-3 content. Marinate the fish briefly in a mixture of lime juice, garlic, and anti-inflammatory spices such as cumin and paprika, then grill or pan-fry until golden and flaky. Serve the fish on soft whole-grain tortillas or lettuce wraps for a lighter option. Accompany these with a slaw made from shredded cabbage, a great source of sulforaphane, an anti-inflammatory compound. Toss the cabbage with carrots and a dressing made from avocado oil, lime juice, and a touch of honey. This combination not only brightens the flavors but also adds a creamy texture without the need for mayonnaise. These tacos are not just delicious; they're also a lively way to enjoy a meal that's good for both your taste buds and your body.

Homemade Pizza Night

Transforming pizza into a healthy meal is easier than you might think. Start with a cauliflower crust, which is lower in carbs and calories than traditional pizza dough and provides a serving of vegetables. Pulse cauliflower in a food processor until fine, steam, and drain well, then mix with an egg, almond flour, and a pinch of salt for binding. Press the mixture into a round shape on a baking sheet and bake until set and starting to brown. For toppings, skip the processed meats and instead layer on antioxidant-rich vegetables like bell peppers, spinach, and tomatoes. Add some grilled chicken for protein and a sprinkle of low-fat mozzarella or nutritional yeast for a cheesy flavor without the excess saturated fat. This pizza is not only a healthier alternative to traditional options but also a fun way for the family to get involved in the cooking process, from shaping the crust to choosing the toppings.

Grill Nights

Grilling is a quintessential part of many family gatherings, and it can be a healthful method of cooking when done right. Choose proteins like fish or chicken, and marinate them in a mix of olive oil, lemon juice, and herbs such as dill or parsley, which are not only flavorful but also offer health benefits. Serve these proteins with grilled vegetables or a side salad for a well-rounded meal. For something a bit different, try making skewers with chunks of salmon, interwoven with slices of zucchini and bell peppers, and a mango salsa on the side. The mango not only adds a sweet, tangy contrast to the savory flavors but also provides a wealth of vitamins and anti-inflammatory compounds.

These weekend meal ideas are designed to bring joy and health to your family gatherings. They show that with a bit of planning and creativity, you can prepare dishes that are loved not only for their flavors but also for the benefits they bring to the table. Enjoy these meals as a way to connect with your loved ones and celebrate the joys of healthy eating.

As we wrap up this chapter on great weekend meals, remember that every dish you prepare is an opportunity to nourish and delight. From the slow-roasted flavors of a family-style roast to the interactive fun of homemade pizza night, these recipes are designed to bring people together and provide nutritious, anti-inflammatory benefits. Carry these ideas into your weekend traditions, making each meal a celebration of good health and great taste. Next, we'll explore how to maintain these healthy eating habits through the seasons, ensuring that you can enjoy vibrant, anti-inflammatory meals all year round.

CHAPTER 4
Meal Planning and Prep

In this chapter, we dive into the art of meal planning, offering you a treasure trove of tips and tricks designed to streamline your cooking process, enhance your diet, and embrace a lifestyle rich in anti-inflammatory foods. Whether you're a seasoned chef or a novice in the kitchen, these guidelines will transform your approach to meal preparation, making it a delightful and health-promoting activity.

4.1 Building a Weekly Meal Plan: Tips and Tricks

Strategic Meal Planning

Embarking on your week with a well-thought-out meal plan can be key for ease and success. It eliminates the guesswork and last-minute decisions that often lead to less healthy choices. Start by envisioning your week—consider your schedule, the time you'll have available each day for cooking, your family schedule, and your energy levels throughout the week. With this overview, begin crafting your meal plan, aiming to balance nutrients each day.

For instance, ensure that each meal includes components from key food groups: a protein source (like beans, fish, or poultry), a good portion of vegetables (the more colorful, the better), a complex carbohydrate (such as quinoa or sweet potatoes), and healthy fats (from sources like avocados or nuts). This not only ensures a well-rounded diet but also helps in managing inflammation, as these food groups are rich in nutrients known to combat inflammatory processes in the body.

Theme Nights

My good friend Shannon had an amazing idea to add an element of fun and predictability to meal planning, consider assigning theme nights. This can simplify decision-making and ensure dietary variety, which is crucial for a balanced diet. For example, designate a "Meatless Monday" to explore plant-based dishes, which are generally low in inflammatory ingredients and rich in nutrients. "Fish Friday" could be your day to enjoy dishes centered around omega-3-rich fish like salmon or mackerel, known for their anti-inflammatory properties. These themed nights not only make planning easier but also ensure that you're incorporating a variety of foods and nutrients into your diet, keeping your meals interesting and health-focused.

Pre-Planning Grocery Lists

Once your meal plan is set, the next step is to create a detailed grocery list. This is a critical step that helps prevent impulse purchases, which often tend to be less healthy options that can derail your dietary goals. Organize your list by categories—produce, proteins, dairy, etc.—to streamline your shopping experience. Check off items you already have in your pantry to avoid duplicates and ensure you buy everything needed for the week's meals. This organized approach not only saves time and money but also supports your commitment to eating a healthful, anti-inflammatory diet throughout the week. Many stores offer grocery pick up for free which can be utilized with these lists to save so much money! No grabbing unnecessary items when someone else does your shopping.

Flexibility in Planning

While a well-structured meal plan is fantastic, life often presents unexpected changes to our schedules. Embracing flexibility within your meal planning can help you adapt without stress. For instance, have a couple of versatile, quick-to-prepare meals up your sleeve for evenings when you're short on time or too tired for a complex recipe. Dishes like stir-fried vegetables and grilled chicken can be whipped up in less than 30 minutes and allow for flexibility in the ingredients, depending on what you have on hand. Similarly, if you find a particular ingredient is unavailable at the store, knowing suitable substitutions can save your meal plan. Spinach can easily substitute for kale, or chickpeas can stand in for lentils, keeping your meals diverse and nutritionally balanced.

Reflective Practice: Weekly Review

At the end of each week, take a moment to reflect on your meals. Which dishes did you enjoy? Which were too time-consuming, and which ingredients didn't hit the mark? This reflection will help you refine your meal planning process, making it more effective and enjoyable each week. Perhaps you'll discover that preparing a large batch of a versatile ingredient like quinoa at the start of the week helped streamline meal prep, or maybe you'll find that you prefer lighter dinners. Use this insight to continuously evolve your meal planning strategy, tailoring it to better meet your dietary needs and preferences, simplifying your cooking routine, and enhancing your overall enjoyment of your meals. In our house, we have a "keep" or "pitch" vote at the end of each meal. If it was a winner dinner, I keep the recipe. If it was a loser, it gets tossed. Then, we always have a pile of beloved recipes tailored to our family's likes and dislikes.

Incorporating strategic meal planning, theme nights, pre-planned grocery lists, and flexibility into your routine sets you up for success in maintaining an anti-inflammatory diet. It makes meal preparation less daunting and more enjoyable, ensuring that you nourish your body with the right foods to combat inflammation and promote overall health. As you move forward, keep refining your approach, adapting it to your evolving needs and preferences, ensuring that each meal is not only a source of nourishment but also a pleasure to prepare and consume.

4.2 Shopping Smart: Budget-Friendly Tips for Anti-Inflammatory Ingredients

Navigating the grocery store or local market can be akin to charting a course through a treasure map, where the gems you're searching for are nutritious, anti-inflammatory foods that don't break the bank. Ugg, that just sounds like a lot of work! Let's break this down into simple, low-stress tips.

One of the smartest strategies you can employ is to focus on seasonal shopping. This method ensures that you're not only getting the freshest and tastiest produce but often at the best prices. Seasonal fruits and vegetables are abundant when they are at their peak, which reduces costs for farmers and distributors, and these savings are passed on to you, the consumer. Moreover, these items are at their nutritional zenith during this time, packed with optimal flavors and anti-inflammatory compounds that can help manage chronic inflammation and boost your overall health.

For example, buying tomatoes in summer or pumpkins in autumn allows you to enjoy these foods when they are most flavorful and nutritious. This practice also encourages a varied diet as you explore different foods available in each season, which is key to a balanced anti-inflammatory diet. Additionally, seasonal foods often require less transportation and storage, reducing their carbon footprint and helping you make more environmentally friendly choices. You might even find that this seasonal approach to shopping rekindles your creativity in the kitchen, inspiring you to try new recipes or revisit traditional ones that celebrate the ingredients of the season.

Another practical approach to smart shopping, especially when you're managing a budget, is buying in bulk. Staples of an anti-inflammatory diet, such as whole grains like quinoa and brown rice or legumes like lentils and chickpeas, are often available in bulk bins. Purchasing these items in larger quantities can significantly lower their cost per serving. Foods bought in bulk can be stored for extended periods if done correctly, ensuring you always have the basics on hand for a variety of meals. This not only saves money but also reduces the frequency of your shopping trips, making it easier to stick to your eating plan without last-minute dashes to the store that could lead to impulse purchases.

Exploring local farmers' markets or joining a community-supported agriculture (CSA) program can further enhance your ability to shop smart. These venues often offer fresh, locally-grown produce at prices comparable to or sometimes cheaper than grocery stores, particularly when you consider the quality and freshness of what you're buying. Farmers' markets also give you a chance to talk directly with growers, learn more about the produce, and sometimes discover new varieties of fruits and vegetables that you might not find in a typical supermarket. Joining a CSA (Community Supported Agriculture) can be a fantastic deal, too. You pay a set fee upfront for a share of the season's harvest, which not only supports local farmers directly but also provides you with regular distributions of fresh produce throughout the growing season.

When it comes to making your diet both cost-effective and anti-inflammatory, knowing how to substitute expensive ingredients with more affordable ones without compromising on nutritional value is crucial. For instance, if a recipe calls for an expensive exotic fruit, look for local fruits that might provide similar nutritional benefits. Similarly, if fresh seafood, which is rich in omega-3 fatty acids, is too pricey, consider canned options like sardines or salmon, which are often cheaper and still offer the same anti-inflammatory benefits. These substitutions not only help keep your meals within budget but also ensure you're adhering to an anti-inflammatory diet by incorporating a variety of nutrients from different sources.

Employing these smart shopping strategies—focusing on seasonal purchases, buying in bulk, exploring local markets, and making cost-effective substitutions—enables you to maintain a rich, diverse anti-inflammatory diet without straining your finances. It empowers you to make choices that benefit your health, support your local economy, and reduce your environmental impact, all while enjoying delicious, nutritious foods that delight your palate.

4.3 Batch Cooking and Freezing for Busy Schedules

The idea of preparing multiple meals in one cooking session might sound daunting at first, but batch cooking is a game-changer for anyone looking to eat healthily without spending hours in the kitchen every day. Imagine spending just a few hours on a Sunday afternoon prepping and cooking, and having a refrigerator and freezer stocked with nutritious meals for the week. This approach not only saves time but also significantly reduces the stress of daily meal preparation, particularly on busy weekdays. By cooking in batches, you're also more likely to stick to your anti-inflammatory diet since you'll have healthy, homemade meals readily available.

When you embark on batch cooking, start by choosing recipes that are both suited to large-scale cooking and meet your dietary needs. Soups, stews, casseroles, and curries are perfect for this. They are not only easy to prepare in large quantities but also tend to freeze well, ensuring that their flavors and nutritional qualities are preserved. For instance, a big pot of vegetable and lentil soup can be a comforting, nutritious meal, and it's easy to make in bulk. Lentils are a fantastic source of protein and fiber and are rich in anti-inflammatory properties, making them an ideal ingredient for your anti-inflammatory diet.

When it comes to preserving the freshness and nutritional integrity of your batch-cooked meals, proper freezing and storage are key. Use airtight containers or heavy-duty freezer bags to store your food, and make sure to label each container with the date and contents. This not only helps in organizing your freezer but also ensures that you use the oldest items first. When filling containers, leave a small space at the top as foods often expand when frozen. This simple step helps prevent the containers from breaking or the lids from popping off.

Sample Batch Cooking Plan

To give you a practical example of how batch cooking can work, let's set up a plan for a week's worth of dinners. On your cooking day, you might prepare a large batch of the aforementioned vegetable and lentil soup, a tray of roasted chicken with mixed vegetables, and a quinoa salad with cherry tomatoes, cucumbers, and a lemon-tahini dressing. Start by preheating your oven for the chicken and vegetables, and while they are roasting, you can cook the lentils and quinoa on the stove. Assemble the salads in individual containers, and once the chicken and vegetables are done, portion them out as well. With these three dishes, you have a variety of meals that provide a balanced array of nutrients and flavors, all prepared in just a few hours.

Thawing and Reheating Best Practices

To enjoy your batch-cooked meals safely and deliciously, proper thawing and reheating are crucial. Always thaw frozen meals in the refrigerator rather than at room temperature to minimize the risk of bacterial growth. Planning ahead is important here; transfer your next day's meal from the freezer to the fridge before going to bed, ensuring it's thawed by the next evening. When reheating, make sure the meal is heated thoroughly until it's steaming hot, which helps kill any potential bacteria. If you're using a microwave, stir the food halfway through heating to ensure it warms evenly.

By incorporating batch cooking and effective freezing techniques into your routine, you can significantly enhance your ability to maintain a healthy, anti-inflammatory diet. It allows you to manage your time efficiently while ensuring that you have access to nutritious meals throughout the week, supporting your health goals without adding to your daily stress. This approach not only simplifies your meal preparation but also frees up more time for you to enjoy other activities, making healthy eating a convenient and enjoyable part of your busy life.

4.4 Quick Fixes: Speedy Solutions for Unexpected Hurdles

Life moves fast, and despite our best intentions, there are days when time just isn't on our side. It's on these days that having a toolkit of quick, healthy recipes can make all the difference, helping you stick to your anti-inflammatory diet without stress or guilt. Let's explore some rapid recipes that you can whip up in no more than 20 minutes, transforming what might have been a mealtime scramble into a delightful, nourishing experience.

For instance, consider the simplicity and speed of a classic avocado and chickpea salad. Begin by slicing a ripe avocado and tossing it with a can of drained chickpeas, a handful of cherry tomatoes, and arugula. Dress this mixture with a quick emulsion of olive oil, lemon juice, a pinch of salt, and a dash of pepper. Not only is this meal quick to prepare, but it's also packed with nutrients such as healthy fats from the avocado and protein from the chickpeas, which are excellent for managing inflammation. Another swift option could be a stir-fry with pre-cut mixed vegetables and a piece of salmon or tofu. Heat a little olive oil in a pan, add the vegetables, and your protein choice, season with a splash of soy sauce and a sprinkle of ginger, and you have a fulfilling dish rich in omega-3 fatty acids and antioxidants in less than 20 minutes.

On the practical side, keeping your kitchen stocked with pre-prepped ingredients can save you precious time. Dedicate a few minutes each weekend to chopping a variety of vegetables and storing them in your fridge. Family shop, chop, and prep time can be a great help AND create healthy habits for young and old alike. Bell peppers, carrots, cucumbers, and broccoli make great options as they can last most of the week when stored properly. Cooked grains like quinoa or brown rice can also be prepared in advance and kept ready for quick assembly during the week. With these ingredients on hand, throwing together a nutritious meal can be as easy as combining some grains, your pre-cut veggies, a protein source like canned beans or baked tofu, and a simple dressing for a quick and easy bowl meal.

Now, even with the best-laid plans, there are days when cooking just isn't in the cards. When you turn to takeout, it's still possible to make anti-inflammatory choices. Opt for dishes rich in vegetables and lean proteins, and be wary of sauces that can be hidden sources of sugar and unhealthy fats. Grilled, steamed, or baked options are usually best. Don't hesitate to ask for modifications—most restaurants are happy to accommodate requests like dressing on the side or substituting a side of fries for a salad. By understanding menu descriptions and not shying away from asking questions about preparation methods, you can enjoy a takeout meal that is both satisfying and aligned with your health goals. My favorite Chinese take-out go-to is steamed chicken and vegetables-no sauce. I can order a large and eat it for a few days. Easy peasy.

Lastly, for those truly hectic days, consider assembling a few emergency meal kits that you can keep in your pantry or freezer. These kits might include a can of no-salt-added beans, pre-cooked rice, a few spices, and some dried vegetables or a jar of preserved veggies. Alternatively, freeze portions of soups, stews, or casseroles that you can quickly reheat. Having these kits on hand means that a wholesome meal is always just minutes away, requiring little to no effort to prepare. This not only ensures you're fed and satisfied on even the busiest days but also keeps you aligned with your dietary goals, effortlessly integrating good nutrition into your fast-paced life. Keep a list on the front of the fridge of these meals, to remind yourself and everyone in the family what's on hand that's fast, prepped, and easy to make.

Each of these strategies—from whipping up quick meals and using pre-prepped ingredients to making smart choices with takeout and creating emergency meal kits—equips you to handle the unexpected twists and turns of everyday life. They ensure that even when time is tight, your commitment to an anti-inflammatory, health-forward diet remains strong and un-compromised. With these tools in your culinary arsenal, you can face the busiest of days with confidence, knowing that a de-licious, nutritious meal is just minutes away, ready to nourish and sustain you no matter the hurdles.

4.5 Integrating Diversity: Catering to All Di-etary Needs

Embracing a diverse range of dietary preferences and needs is not just about inclusivity; it's about ensuring that everyone at your table can enjoy delicious, health-promoting meals regard-less of their dietary restrictions or cultural background. This becomes especially important when adopting an anti-inflam-matory diet, as the broader the variety of foods you can incor-porate, the more balanced and effective your diet will be. Let's explore how you can adapt your meal planning to accommo-date a wide array of dietary needs, making your meals a source of comfort and health for everyone involved.

For those with food allergies or sensitivities, navigating meal plans can often feel restrictive. Common allergens like nuts, dairy, and gluten not only appear in obvious places but also hide in less-expected foods, making meal preparation a challenge. However, with a few smart substitutions, you can create dishes that are safe and enjoyable for everyone. Instead of peanut butter, for instance, consider seed butters like sunflower or pumpkin seed butter, which can provide a similar creamy texture and nutritional benefits without the allergen risk. For dairy alternatives, coconut milk, and oat milk offer rich textures and are generally well-tolerated by those who are lactose intolerant or allergic to cow's milk. In the realm of gluten-free cooking, almond flour, and chickpea flour are excellent for baking and cooking, providing high protein content and a pleasing texture without the gluten.

Incorporating a variety of culturally diverse recipes not only enriches your culinary repertoire but also respects and celebrates the cultural backgrounds of those you cook for. Dishes like Moroccan tagine, which uses a plethora of spices like turmeric and cinnamon, can offer potent anti-inflammatory benefits while providing a taste of North African cuisine. Similarly, a traditional Indian dal made from lentils and spiced with cumin and mustard seeds offers a comforting, nutritious meal that adheres to anti-inflammatory principles while catering to vegetarian preferences. These dishes not only broaden your culinary horizons but also ensure that your diet remains interesting and varied, key components in maintaining long-term adherence to an anti-inflammatory eating plan.

Vegetarian and vegan diets are increasingly popular, both for health and ethical reasons, and they naturally align well with anti-inflammatory eating principles due to their emphasis on plant-based foods. To ensure that your meal plans are vegetarian or vegan-friendly while still adhering to anti-inflammatory guidelines, focus on including a variety of plant-based proteins like beans, lentils, and tofu. These ingredients can be wonderfully versatile, fitting seamlessly into a range of dishes from different cuisines. For example, tofu can be marinated and used in stir-fries, salads, or even grilled, providing a satisfying protein source that is both vegan and anti-inflammatory. Beans and lentils can be turned into hearty soups, spicy curries, or refreshing salads, providing ample opportunities to vary your meals while keeping them plant-based and inflammation-friendly.

When planning meals for a family or group with varying age groups and activity levels, it's important to tailor your meals to meet the different nutritional needs. Children and teenagers, for instance, have higher energy needs and might require more carbohydrates and proteins, which can be provided through dishes like whole-grain pasta with a bean-based sauce or a quinoa salad packed with chopped vegetables and seeds. Older adults, on the other hand, might require fewer calories but more of certain nutrients like calcium and vitamin D, which can be incorporated through foods like fortified plant milks and leafy green vegetables. One of my biggest pet peeves in practice was for older adults to try to get calcium from milk. The most bang for your buck nutritionally is going to come from leafy green vegetables. Far better to use them to build strong bones gradually over time than to wait and need a medication that tends to build Phosphorus bones, which aren't as strong and durable. For those with higher activity levels, incorporating more protein-rich snacks or meals, like smoothies with hemp seeds or chicken breast strips with a quinoa and vegetable mix, can help in muscle repair and energy replenishment. By considering these factors, you ensure that your meal plans are not only anti-inflammatory and inclusive but also fine-tuned to nurture the health of all who gather at your table, regardless of their age or activity level.

Through thoughtful consideration of allergies, cultural preferences, dietary choices, and individual nutritional needs, your approach to meal planning can be both comprehensive and compassionate. This attentiveness ensures that your meals are not just nourishing but also welcoming to everyone, making your dining table a place of health and community. As you continue to explore and integrate these principles into your culinary practices, remember that every meal is an opportunity to nurture, delight, and bring people together, creating not just delicious dishes but also fostering well-being and harmony among those you care for.

4.6 Seasonal Eating: Maximizing Fresh, Local Produce

As briefly mentioned above, eating seasonally is one of those delightful approaches that harmoniously blends the pleasure of tasting the freshest produce with the practical benefits of nutritional gain and cost savings. When you choose fruits and vegetables that are in their peak season, you're not only enjoying produce at its most flavorful but also at its nutritional zenith. Seasonal produce tends to be richer in vitamins and antioxidants—the compounds that play a crucial role in reducing inflammation and enhancing overall health. These nutrients are at their highest when fruits and vegetables are harvested at the right time, offering you the best in flavor and health benefits.

For instance, consider the vibrant strawberries of early summer or the robust butternut squash in fall. These not only bring a burst of flavor to your meals but are also packed with vitamins, minerals, and other anti-inflammatory compounds that can help combat chronic health issues. Eating these foods shortly after harvest means the nutrients are more intact compared to out-of-season produce that may have traveled long distances and been stored for long periods, gradually losing their nutritional value.

To effectively incorporate seasonal eating into your lifestyle, a seasonal food chart can be immensely helpful. This tool guides you on what produce to look for at different times of the year, ensuring you can plan your meals around the freshest, most nutritious options available. For spring, focus on greens such as asparagus and peas, which can add crispness and vibrancy to your meals. Summer offers a bounty of options like berries, cucumbers, and tomatoes, perfect for light salads or refreshing desserts. In autumn, turn to hearty squashes and root vegetables, which are excellent for warm soups and roasts. Winter calls for citrus fruits and leafy greens, which can brighten up darker days with their nutrients and flavors.

Incorporating these seasonal foods into your daily meals can be both exciting and beneficial. In spring, a simple salad of mixed greens, including fresh peas and asparagus with a lemon vinaigrette, can be both cleansing and invigorating. Summer might see you blending berries with yogurt for a cooling smoothie or tossing together a tomato and cucumber salad with a drizzle of olive oil and herbs. When fall arrives, a squash soup seasoned with ginger can warm you up and boost your immune system. Winter citrus fruits are perfect for adding a tangy punch to dark leafy greens in salads or for brightening up a winter stew.

Preserving seasonal produce allows you to extend these benefits throughout the year. Methods like canning, drying, or pickling not only save the bounty of the season but also ensure you have access to healthy ingredients that retain most of their beneficial properties. Canning tomatoes or making berry jams can provide you with delightful, healthful options that are far superior to store-bought versions often laden with additives. Drying herbs or making your own dried fruit like apple chips or apricots offers wonderful, preservative-free snack options. Pickling vegetables such as cucumbers or carrots can also add a flavorful, nutritious kick to meals.

By embracing the rhythm of the seasons, you not only enrich your diet in a way that is aligned with nature but also support local agriculture and reduce your ecological footprint. This approach to eating not only brings variety and freshness into your meals but also helps you engage with your food on a deeper level, understanding where it comes from and how it contributes to your health.

As you continue to explore the rich tapestry of seasonal eating, remember that each season brings its own flavors and health benefits. Integrating this practice into your life isn't just about enjoying fresher, tastier food—it's about making choices that enhance your health, support your local community, and respect the environment. This chapter hopefully provides you with the knowledge and inspiration to fully embrace seasonal eating, enriching your diet and your life with every changing season.

Reflecting on the Journey Through Seasonal Eating

As this chapter closes, we've traveled through the vibrant world of seasonal eating, exploring how aligning your diet with the cycles of nature can enrich your health and palate. From understanding the nutritional peaks of seasonal produce to integrating these gems into your everyday meals and preserving their goodness to enjoy year-round, you've gained insights into making the most of what each season offers. As you move forward, carry with you the knowledge that with each season's turn, a new bounty awaits, ready to enhance your meals and your health.

If you are enjoying this book, please stop and leave us a review!

Reviews are how others hear about which books out there are worth the read. Please help us spread the word today via Amazon.com!

CHAPTER 5
Beyond Diet—Lifestyle Factors Influencing Inflammation

Embracing an anti-inflammatory lifestyle extends beyond the kitchen and into the very movements of your daily life. Think of your body as a finely tuned instrument; just as a guitar needs strumming to resonate melodies, your body requires movement to maintain its harmony. Physical activity, an essential melody in the symphony of your well-being, not only tunes your cardiovascular health but also plays a critical role in moderating inflammatory responses. Let's explore how integrating regular physical activity into your routine can be a profound melody that brings wellness into your life, particularly in reducing inflammation.

5.1 The Role of Physical Activity in Reducing Inflammation

Mechanisms of Action

Physical activity, in its various forms, acts like a balm, soothing the chronic inflammation that can lead to numerous health issues. When you engage in regular exercise, your body responds not just with increased fitness but also with biological changes at the cellular level. Exercise stimulates the production of macrophages, a type of white blood cell that helps reduce inflammation by clearing out inflammatory cells. Moreover, it leads to the release of cytokines, proteins that are crucial in the immune system, which include types that help reduce inflammation. When you exercise, the levels of pro-inflammatory cytokines decrease, while anti-inflammatory cytokines increase, creating a more balanced immune response. Regular physical activity also helps in lowering levels of C-reactive protein, a substance produced by the liver in response to inflammation, commonly used as a marker to assess inflammation levels in the body.

Recommended Types of Exercise

Incorporating a mix of aerobic activities, strength training, and flexibility exercises create a comprehensive exercise regimen that can help manage and reduce inflammation. Aerobic exercises, such as brisk walking, cycling, or swimming, increase your heart rate and improve your cardiovascular health, which is crucial for reducing inflammation. Strength training, on the other hand, builds muscle mass, which is important not only for overall strength but also for regulating insulin levels and stimulating anti-inflammatory chemicals in the body. Flexibility exercises, such as yoga or tai chi, not only improve your range of motion and reduce stress but also have been shown to lower inflammatory markers, particularly in those with chronic diseases like rheumatoid arthritis.

Creating a Balanced Exercise Routine

To keep your exercise routine enjoyable and effective, variety is key. Imagine crafting a weekly schedule that includes a mix of walking, yoga sessions, and perhaps a dance class. This variety not only keeps boredom at bay but also allows different muscle groups to engage and recover, minimizing the risk of injury. Start with activities you enjoy, as the pleasure derived from exercise can be a powerful motivator. Gradually increase the duration and intensity to avoid overwhelming your body and to keep the challenge fresh. Remember, consistency is more critical than intensity when starting out. Aim for at least 150 minutes of moderate aerobic activity or 75 minutes of vigorous activity each week, as recommended by health guidelines, and include muscle-strengthening activities on two or more days a week. Having a workout buddy always makes things more fun too.

Case Studies and Research

The link between regular physical activity and reduced inflammation is not just theoretical but is backed by numerous studies. For instance, a research study published in the "Journal of the American Heart Association" found that middle-aged individuals who engaged in regular physical activity had significantly lower levels of inflammation markers, including C-reactive protein and interleukin-6, compared to those who were inactive. Another compelling case is that of a 52-year-old patient, Kathleen, who, after incorporating 30 minutes of moderate exercise into her daily routine, saw a marked improvement in her inflammatory markers and overall health within just six months! These real-life examples underscore the transformative power of physical activity in managing inflammation and enhancing quality of life.

Physical activity, therefore, is not merely about keeping fit or losing weight; it's a fundamental part of managing inflammation and maintaining health. As you lace up your sneakers or unroll your yoga mat, remember that each step, each stretch, each lift is a step toward a less inflamed you. Whether you're taking a brisk walk in the morning sunshine or lifting weights in the cool of your living room, your body is getting tuned up, inflammation is getting toned down, and your overall health is playing a better tune.

5.2 Sleep's Impact on Inflammation and How to Improve Your Sleep Hygiene

The silent hours of the night offer more than just a pause from the bustling activities of daytime; they are a crucial time for your body to repair and rejuvenate. This nightly renewal is deeply intertwined with your immune system's function, particularly how it handles inflammation. Poor sleep quality or insufficient sleep can disrupt this process, leading to increased inflammation. During sleep, your body produces cytokines, which are proteins that help regulate inflammation and immunity. If sleep is cut short or is of poor quality, production of these protective cytokines diminishes, while inflammatory markers increase. This imbalance can exacerbate existing inflammatory conditions like arthritis or even increase the risk of developing new inflammatory issues.

Tips for Better Sleep Hygiene

To harness the healing power of sleep, establishing a sound sleep hygiene routine is essential. First and foremost, maintaining a regular sleep schedule can significantly improve the quality of your rest. Going to bed and waking up at the same time every day sets your body's internal clock to expect rest at certain hours, improving your chances of falling asleep quickly and enjoying deep, restorative sleep.

Creating a restful environment also plays a crucial role in combating sleep-related inflammation. Your bedroom should be a sanctuary designed to promote relaxation and comfort. Invest in a good quality mattress and pillows that support your body and align with your sleeping position. Ensure your room is dark, quiet, and cool—conditions that signal to your body it's time to wind down. Consider blackout curtains, earplugs, or a white noise machine to block out disruptions. Additionally, the blue light emitted by screens can interfere with your body's natural sleep-wake cycle. Limiting screen time for at least an hour before bed can help your mind unwind and prepare for sleep.

Tools and Technologies

In today's tech-savvy world, various tools and technologies can assist you in achieving better sleep. Sleep trackers, either standalone devices or features within fitness trackers, can provide insights into your sleep patterns, helping you understand what helps or hinders your sleep quality. These devices typically monitor movements and heart rate to estimate different sleep stages, from light and deep sleep to REM cycles, offering data that can help you tweak your sleep habits for the better.

White noise machines are another valuable tool, particularly for those who find themselves easily awakened by background noise. By producing consistent, soothing sounds, these machines can mask disruptive noises such as traffic or loud neighbors, creating a more controlled and calming auditory environment that promotes better sleep.

Impact of Sleep Disorders

Recognizing and addressing sleep disorders is crucial as they can significantly impact inflammation and overall health. Conditions like sleep apnea, where breathing repeatedly stops and starts throughout the night, can severely disrupt sleep and increase stress and inflammation in the body. People with untreated sleep apnea often experience elevated levels of C-reactive protein and other inflammatory markers, linking directly to an increased risk of cardiovascular and other systemic diseases.

If you suspect a sleep disorder, consult your healthcare provider. Treatments may include lifestyle changes, such as weight loss and smoking cessation, or medical interventions like CPAP machines or oral appliances, which can dramatically improve sleep quality and reduce inflammatory responses in the body.

Integrating these practices—tailoring your sleep environment, regulating sleep schedules, using technological aids, and addressing sleep disorders—can transform your nights into a powerful tool against inflammation. As you lay down tonight, remember that each hour of restful sleep is a step towards a healthier, less inflamed tomorrow.

5.3 Stress Reduction Techniques That Work

Stress often acts as a silent catalyst for inflammation, weaving its effects subtly yet significantly through your body. When you experience chronic stress, your body's fight-or-flight response is triggered, releasing a cascade of stress hormones like cortisol and adrenaline. These hormones, while beneficial in short bursts, can lead to increased blood pressure and a higher production of inflammatory cytokines when continuously present. This hormonal imbalance not only disrupts your body's normal processes but also exacerbates conditions linked to inflammation, such as arthritis, heart disease, and asthma. Understanding this connection highlights the importance of managing stress not just for mental well-being but also as a crucial element in controlling inflammation.

To effectively manage and mitigate stress, various techniques can be employed, each with its own method of calming the mind and reducing the physical impacts of stress. Mindfulness meditation is one such powerful practice. It involves sitting quietly and paying attention to thoughts, sounds, the sensations of breathing, or parts of the body, bringing your attention back whenever the mind starts to wander. Practicing mindfulness meditation can help you become more aware of your thoughts and feelings so that instead of being overwhelmed by them, you're better able to manage them. Engaging in this practice regularly can lower levels of cortisol, thereby reducing the inflammatory response associated with chronic stress.

Deep breathing exercises are another simple yet effective method to reduce stress. Techniques such as diaphragmatic breathing, which involves deep, even breaths from the diaphragm rather than shallow breaths from the chest, can help reduce heart rate and promote relaxation. This type of breathing helps to activate the body's relaxation response, shifting the balance from the stress response to a more calm, restful state. Even a few minutes of deep breathing can have a significant impact, making this a useful technique for quick stress relief in any setting.

Progressive muscle relaxation (PMR) is another technique that can be particularly effective in alleviating stress. It involves tensing each muscle group in the body tightly, but not to the point of strain, and then slowly relaxing them. This practice promotes awareness of physical sensations and helps in the gradual relaxation of the entire body. By focusing on the release of physical tension, PMR can also help to ease mental tension, as the state of the body often affects the state of the mind. Mind over matter.

Integrating these stress reduction practices into your daily routine can significantly enhance their benefits. Set aside a specific time each day for mindfulness meditation, even if it's just five minutes in the morning. This helps to establish it as a habit and reinforces its importance in your daily life. Keeping a journal can also be useful. After each session, jot down any changes in your stress level or how you physically feel. This can help you identify which techniques are most effective for you and encourage you to continue practicing. For deep breathing and PMR, consider using transitions between different parts of your day—such as after work or before bed—as cues for these exercises. This not only ensures regular practice but also helps in managing stress promptly, preventing it from accumulating and bubbling over.

The personal stories of those who have incorporated these techniques into their lives speak volumes about their effectiveness. Consider the example of a middle-aged professional, Annie, who began practicing mindfulness meditation regularly. Over several months, not only did her daily stress levels decrease, but follow-up medical tests also showed a significant reduction in markers of inflammation. Her experience underscores the potential of these techniques to transform not just mental health but also physical health by moderating the body's inflammatory responses. Her family was so excited to have a much more relaxed Mom too.

Embracing these techniques, understanding their benefits, and making them a part of your daily life can open up a path to enhanced well-being and reduced inflammation. Each method offers a unique approach to managing stress, providing you with a toolkit of options to maintain your health in the face of life's inevitable pressures. As you continue to explore and apply these strategies, remember that the goal is not to eliminate stress entirely but to manage it so effectively that it no longer controls your health or your happiness.

5.4 Hydration and Its Underrated Role in Managing Inflammation

Water is the essence of life, yet its pivotal role in managing inflammation and maintaining overall health often goes unnoticed. Every cell, tissue, and organ in your body needs water to work properly. From serving as a primary component of saliva for digestion to regulating your body temperature through sweating, water is indispensable. Furthermore, adequate hydration helps in the elimination of waste through urine, carries nutrients and oxygen to cells, and cushions joints. When it comes to inflammation, staying well-hydrated is crucial because it helps to flush out toxins and other waste materials from the body, which can trigger or worsen inflammation. Moreover, adequate hydration ensures that your blood maintains a consistency that allows it to flow freely, transporting various anti-inflammatory compounds to where they are needed and facilitating the removal of pro-inflammatory agents effectively.

Navigating how much water you should consume daily can sometimes feel like a complex calculus, but it doesn't have to be. The amount of water required can vary based on several factors including your age, sex, activity level, and the climate you live in. Generally, a good rule of thumb for adults is to drink at least 1/2 of your body weight in ounces a day. However, if you lead a particularly active lifestyle or reside in a hot climate, your body will likely require additional hydration to compensate for the increased fluid loss through sweat. It's also important to adjust your water intake based on your body's signals. Feeling thirsty, for instance, is a clear indication that your body may need more fluids. Be cautious to balance water with electrolytes on hot days as well.

Recognizing the signs of dehydration is critical, as even mild dehydration can exacerbate inflammatory responses and interfere with your body's normal functions. Common indicators include thirst, infrequent urination, dark-colored urine, fatigue, dizziness, and dry skin. If you notice these signs, it's a signal to increase your fluid intake. To ensure consistent hydration throughout the day, carrying a water bottle can be remarkably effective. Make a habit of sipping from it regularly, and refill it several times a day. Glasses with straws make sipping easier on the go. If you find plain water too bland, adding slices of fruits like lemon, lime, or cucumber can enhance the flavor, making it more appealing and encouraging you to drink more.

In addition to drinking water, you can boost your hydration levels through your diet. Many fruits and vegetables are high in water content and can contribute significantly to your daily hydration needs. Foods like cucumbers, celery, and watermelon are not only refreshing but are over 90% water, making them excellent choices for staying hydrated. These foods also bring a bounty of anti-inflammatory benefits, thanks to their high content of antioxidants and other beneficial compounds. Including a variety of these hydrating foods in your meals and snacks can help maintain optimal hydration levels and reduce inflammation. For instance, starting your day with a breakfast that includes watermelon or adding slices of cucumber to your water or your salad at lunch can be simple yet effective strategies to enhance your hydration and your health.

As you continue to navigate your day-to-day activities, remember that maintaining adequate hydration is a simple yet powerful tool for managing inflammation and enhancing your overall well-being. Whether through the water you drink or the foods you choose, each sip and bite is an opportunity to nourish your body, combat inflammation, and move closer to a state of optimal health. Keep your water bottle close, enjoy hydrating foods, and listen to your body's needs to keep inflammation at bay and your body functioning at its best.

5.5 The Importance of Gut Health in Controlling Inflammation

The bustling metropolis of microorganisms residing within your gut, known as the gut microbiome, plays a pivotal role in your overall health, particularly in how your body manages inflammation. This complex network of bacteria, fungi, and viruses significantly influences the immune system, which in turn affects inflammatory responses throughout the body. When your gut microbiome is balanced and healthy, it supports the immune system in functioning efficiently, helping to prevent excessive or inappropriate inflammatory responses that can lead to chronic diseases. Conversely, an imbalance in this microbiome—a condition known as dysbiosis—can trigger increased gut permeability, commonly referred to as "leaky gut," where bacteria and toxins leak through intestinal walls, triggering inflammation and potentially leading to various chronic conditions.

The interaction between the gut microbiome and the immune system is a fine dance of complex biological processes. Beneficial bacteria in the gut produce short-chain fatty acids through the fermentation of dietary fibers, which not only serve as energy sources for colon cells but also modulate immune responses, enhancing the body's anti-inflammatory pathways. These beneficial microbes also help in the production of certain types of cytokines that regulate the immune system's response to disease and infection, ensuring that inflammatory responses are appropriate and not overly aggressive, which can lead to auto-immune diseases.

To foster a healthy gut microbiome, the roles of probiotics and prebiotics are indispensable. Probiotics are live bacteria found in certain yogurts, supplements, and fermented foods like sauerkraut, kimchi, and kefir. These beneficial microorganisms can help restore the natural balance of your gut bacteria, enhancing digestion and immune function, and subsequently reducing inflammatory responses. Prebiotics, on the other hand, are types of dietary fiber that feed the friendly bacteria in your digestive system. Found in foods such as bananas, onions, garlic, leeks, asparagus, and whole grains, prebiotics help beneficial bacteria flourish, promoting a balanced gut microbiome and supporting the immune system in its role of managing inflammation.

Recognizing signs of poor gut health is crucial for taking timely action to mitigate inflammation. Common symptoms that may indicate an unhealthy gut include frequent bloating, gas, constipation, diarrhea, and irregular bowel movements. These symptoms can be signs that your gut microbiome is imbalanced, leading to ineffective digestion and absorption of nutrients, which can trigger inflammatory responses in the body. If you experience these symptoms regularly, it might be time to evaluate your diet and lifestyle to incorporate more probiotic and prebiotic-rich foods, which can help rebalance your gut flora, enhance your digestive health, and reduce inflammation.

Specific dietary adjustments can further promote a healthier gut microbiome and therefore help control inflammation. Integrating a diverse range of fibrous foods into your diet is important. Fiber serves as a primary fuel source for beneficial gut bacteria, and a varied fiber intake promotes a diverse microbiome, which is associated with better health outcomes. Include a variety of fibrous foods such as legumes, beans, berries, whole grains, and leafy greens in your meals. Additionally, the inclusion of fermented foods rich in probiotics not only supports gut health but also adds new flavors and textures to your diet, making meals more interesting.

Your gut health plays a foundational role in managing inflammation and overall wellness. By understanding and nurturing the gut-immune system interaction through appropriate dietary choices and lifestyle habits, you can enjoy not only improved gut health but also enhanced systemic health and reduced risk of inflammation-related conditions. Encouraging the growth of beneficial gut bacteria with a diet rich in diverse fibers and fermented foods, being mindful of symptoms that indicate gut imbalance, and taking steps to address these can lead to significant improvements in your quality of life and health.

5.6 Holistic Approaches: Supplements and Natural Remedies

In your quest to live a life with less inflammation, you might find a valuable ally in the world of supplements and natural remedies. These potent aids can enhance your diet and lifestyle choices, helping to manage and reduce inflammation more effectively. For instance, turmeric, mentioned quite a few times here already and known for its active compound curcumin, has been celebrated for its potent anti-inflammatory properties. Regular supplementation with turmeric can help reduce the pain associated with inflammatory conditions like arthritis, thanks to curcumin's ability to inhibit key enzymes in the inflammation pathway. However, curcumin is not easily absorbed by the body, so it's often recommended to take it with black pepper, which contains Piperine, a natural substance that enhances the absorption of curcumin by up to 2000%.

Omega-3 fatty acids, found abundantly in fish oil, flaxseeds, and walnuts, are another cornerstone of anti-inflammatory supplementation and are worth mentioning again. These fats are crucial in building the structures of cell membranes and are powerful anti-inflammatories that help regulate the body's inflammation cycles. Regular intake of omega-3 supplements can significantly reduce the cytokine levels in the body, lowering inflammation and potentially reducing the risk of chronic diseases such as heart disease and diabetes. It's important to choose high-quality omega-3 supplements and to consult with a healthcare provider to determine the right dosage.

Ginger, another powerful anti-inflammatory, can be taken in various forms such as capsules, teas, or fresh root. This versatile supplement helps reduce inflammation by inhibiting the synthesis of pro-inflammatory cytokines and chemokines in the body. Beyond its benefits for reducing inflammation, ginger can also alleviate nausea and enhance immune function, making it a wonderful addition to your daily regimen.

Turning to herbal remedies, green tea is acclaimed not only for its ability to enhance alertness and mood but also for its high levels of epigallocatechin gallate (EGCG), a natural antioxidant that can help fight inflammation. Drinking green tea daily can significantly reduce the markers of inflammation and protect against certain chronic diseases. Ashwagandha, an herb commonly used in Ayurvedic medicine, is known for its adaptogenic properties that help the body manage stress, a common cause of inflammation. Regular consumption of ashwagandha can help to modulate the body's response to stress and reduce the levels of cortisol, thus indirectly reducing inflammation.

Boswellia, also known as Indian frankincense, contains active components like boswellic acids that are potent anti-inflammatories. These compounds can prevent the formation of leukotrienes, molecules that can cause inflammation. Boswellia is particularly effective in reducing inflammation associated with osteoarthritis and rheumatoid arthritis, often improving symptoms and increasing mobility.

While these supplements and herbal remedies can be powerful tools in managing inflammation, safety should always be your top priority. It is crucial to consult with a healthcare provider before starting any new supplement or natural remedy, especially if you are taking other medications or have underlying health conditions. This step ensures that you avoid any potential interactions and that your supplement regimen is safe and effective. For instance, supplements like omega-3 fatty acids can interact with blood-thinning medications, and some ingredients in herbal remedies might exacerbate certain health conditions.

In addition to these supplements and remedies, consider exploring integrative practices like acupuncture and massage therapy, which can further enhance your anti-inflammatory efforts. Acupuncture, a traditional Chinese medical practice, involves inserting thin needles into specific points on the body. This can help improve blood flow and reduce muscle tension, thereby reducing inflammation and promoting relaxation. Massage therapy, on the other hand, can increase circulation and lymph flow, helping to flush out inflammatory toxins from the tissues.

As you integrate these holistic approaches into your lifestyle, remember that they are most effective when used in conjunction with a balanced diet and a healthy lifestyle. Supplements and natural remedies can provide additional support, helping you achieve a more comprehensive approach to managing inflammation.

Reflecting on Holistic Approaches to Reducing Inflammation

This exploration of holistic approaches underscores the powerful role that supplements, natural remedies, and integrative practices can play in managing inflammation. From the potent anti-inflammatory effects of turmeric and omega-3 fatty acids to the stress-reducing properties of ashwagandha and the physical benefits of acupuncture and massage therapy, these strategies offer a multi-faceted approach to enhancing your health.

Looking ahead, the next chapter will build on these foundational strategies, exploring advanced topics in managing inflammation. This will include cutting-edge research, innovative treatments, and emerging trends in the field of inflammation management, providing you with the knowledge and tools to continue refining your approach to health and wellness.

CHAPTER 6
Overcoming Challenges and Staying Motivated

Imagine standing at a buffet filled with a dazzling array of dishes, each more tempting than the last. Now, imagine that you are there not just to enjoy this feast but to make choices that favor your health, specifically anti-inflammatory choices that support your well-being. This scenario isn't just about food; it's a metaphor for the daily decisions and interactions you face as you adhere to an anti-inflammatory lifestyle. It's about navigating social settings without feeling restricted, and enjoying life's pleasures while maintaining your health goals. This chapter is dedicated to helping you manage one of the most common challenges: dining socially, whether at restaurants or parties, without losing track of your dietary objectives.

6.1 Handling Social Dining: Eating Out and Parties

When it comes to dining out or celebrating at social gatherings, the key to maintaining your anti-inflammatory diet without feeling like you're missing out lies in making informed choices and planning. Start by becoming a savvy menu reader. Most restaurants now offer a range of healthy options, but the trick is to know what to look for. Opt for dishes that are rich in vegetables and lean proteins, as these are staples of an anti-inflammatory diet. Grilled salmon, for example, is not only delicious but also packed with omega-3 fatty acids, which are excellent for fighting inflammation. Vegetarian dishes that feature legumes, whole grains, and a colorful array of vegetables are also great choices.

However, it's not just about what you choose to eat, but also how it's prepared. Sauces and dressings can be hidden sources of unhealthy fats and sugars, which can provoke inflammation. Always ask for dressings and sauces to be served on the side. This simple strategy allows you to control the amount you consume, or even skip them altogether if they don't meet your dietary needs. Don't hesitate to ask how the food is prepared. Opt for cooking methods that require less fat, such as steaming, grilling, or baking, rather than fried foods.

Communication with restaurant staff or your host at a party is crucial. Don't shy away from discussing your dietary restrictions. Most chefs and hosts are more than willing to accommodate your needs, especially if you communicate clearly and respectfully. Explain that you are following an anti-inflammatory diet and specify what ingredients you need to avoid. This open dialogue not only ensures that your dietary needs are met but also raises awareness about the importance of offering healthy, anti-inflammatory options.

Planning ahead is another effective strategy to ensure you stick to your anti-inflammatory goals while dining out. Most restaurants offer their menus online, providing you the perfect opportunity to peruse the options at your leisure and plan your meal ahead of time. This prevents the all-too-common stress of making a hurried decision at the table, which can lead to less healthy choices. If you're attending a party, consider offering to bring a dish. This not only guarantees that there will be at least one anti-inflammatory option available, but it also shows your host that you're proactive and considerate.

Balancing flexibility and commitment is perhaps the most delicate part of managing your diet in social settings. It's important to remember that strict adherence to any diet can sometimes lead to feelings of deprivation or social isolation, which are not conducive to overall well-being. Allow yourself the flexibility to indulge occasionally in foods that might not strictly fall within the anti-inflammatory category, especially during special occasions. The key is moderation. Enjoy a small portion of that birthday cake or a special holiday dish. Such indulgences, when enjoyed mindfully and occasionally, can enhance your enjoyment of social events without significantly derailing your dietary goals.

Navigating social dining successfully is about making informed choices, communicating your needs, and planning, but it's also about balance. By mastering these strategies, you ensure that your social life and your health goals are not at odds but are instead complementary parts of a fulfilling, healthy lifestyle. Whether you're at a summer barbecue, a cozy winter dinner party, or dining out at your favorite restaurant, you can enjoy the pleasures of good food and good company while staying committed to your anti-inflammatory diet. Remember, every meal is an opportunity to nourish not just your body, but also your relationships and your joy in life.

6.2 What If You Slip? Managing Diet Missteps

You've been diligently following your anti-inflammatory diet, enjoying the vibrant colors and diverse flavors of nutritious foods, and feeling proud of your commitment. Then, one evening at a friend's birthday celebration, you indulge in a slice of chocolate cake—a choice that strays from your dietary plan. When this happens, remember, that slipping up is a natural part of any lifestyle change, not a failure. Embracing this as a moment of learning rather than a setback can transform your approach to maintaining your diet in the long run.

Firstly, understand that perfection is not the goal; resilience and consistency are. One slip does not undo all the progress you have made. It's important to avoid harsh self-criticism or guilt, which can lead to more stress and potentially more inflammatory responses in your body. Instead, take a moment to reflect on what led to this choice. Was it the social pressure, a lack of planning, or simply the desire to indulge? Acknowledging the triggers helps you prepare strategies to handle similar situations in the future. For instance, if noticing that social settings often lead to dietary slips, you might decide to eat a healthy meal before attending events to avoid temptation or bring your own anti-inflammatory dish to share, ensuring there's something you can enjoy without guilt.

Constructive responses are key. Rather than dwelling on the misstep, focus on what you can learn from the experience. Each slip provides valuable insights into your dietary habits and triggers. Use this knowledge to strengthen your resolve and refine your strategy. Perhaps you'll discover the need for more varied meals within your diet to reduce feelings of deprivation, or maybe you'll find that keeping healthy snacks on hand can prevent choices made out of hunger. Documenting these reflections can be incredibly helpful, whether in a journal or a digital app, as it allows you to track patterns over time and make adjustments based on real experiences.

Moreover, the speed at which you reset after a slip-up impacts your long-term success. Instead of letting one off-choice lead you down a path of unhealthy eating, return to your anti-inflammatory diet at the next meal. This quick reset helps reinforce your commitment to your health goals and prevents the common mindset of "I've already messed up, I might as well continue." Every meal is a new opportunity to nourish your body in alignment with your health objectives.

Lastly, maintaining perspective is crucial. It's easy to get caught up in daily fluctuations, but the bigger picture is what truly matters. Your overall health and well-being are built over time, through a series of choices that, collectively, create your lifestyle. Consistent, long-term habits have a far more significant impact on your health than occasional deviations. This perspective helps you focus on progress rather than perfection, fostering a more forgiving and sustainable approach to dietary management.

Navigating your dietary choices, particularly when transitioning to an anti-inflammatory lifestyle, is akin to steering a boat on a vast ocean. There will be waves and there will be calm, but each day you learn a little more about how to sail smoothly. Remember, it's not about never falling overboard; it's about knowing how to swim back to your boat and continue your voyage. Embrace each slip as part of your journey, learn from it, and let it guide you to a healthier, more informed place.

6.3 Finding Support and Community Online and Offline

Embarking on an anti-inflammatory lifestyle can sometimes feel like a solitary endeavor, but it doesn't have to be. In fact, finding a community of like-minded individuals can be one of the most uplifting parts of this process. Whether online or in person, connecting with others who are also committed to reducing inflammation through diet and lifestyle changes can provide not just support and motivation, but also a wealth of shared knowledge and experiences.

Online platforms have revolutionized the way we connect, and they offer an expansive range of options for anyone seeking support on their health journey. Social media groups, dedicated health forums, and blogs focused on anti-inflammatory living can be valuable resources. These platforms allow you to share your experiences, challenges, and successes while learning from others. For instance, Facebook and Reddit have numerous groups dedicated to anti-inflammatory diets where members regularly post meal ideas, share scientific articles, and offer emotional support. Engaging with these communities can help you feel less isolated, more understood, and significantly more empowered.

Moreover, many health and wellness influencers on platforms like Instagram and YouTube share their personal journeys and professional advice about living an anti-inflammatory lifestyle. Following these accounts can not only provide daily inspiration but also practical tips that can be easily incorporated into your routine. Additionally, these platforms often host live sessions where you can ask questions and interact directly with experts and community members, making the support even more personal and immediate.

However, while online platforms are wonderfully accessible, the value of face-to-face interactions should not be underestimated. Local support groups or wellness circles can offer a different kind of connection. Many community centers, health clinics, and even some libraries host regular meetings for people interested in topics like anti-inflammatory diets, where you can meet and interact with peers in your area. These meetings often feature talks from guest speakers, including nutritionists and healthcare providers, who can provide professional guidance and answer questions in real time.

Involving your friends and family in your anti-inflammatory lifestyle can also enhance your support system. Start by sharing what you've learned about how inflammation affects health and how diet can play a key role in managing it. This not only educates them but might also pique their interest in joining you or supporting your dietary choices. Invite them to participate in meal planning and preparation. This not only makes the process more fun but also easier to manage. Cooking together can be a bonding activity, and it helps others appreciate the richness and variety of an anti-inflammatory diet.

Furthermore, don't hesitate to seek out professional guidance if needed. Lifelong Metabolic Center is here to help. We can offer personalized advice based on your specific health needs and goals. For instance, we can help you reset your metabolism using an anti-inflammatory and low glycemic plan followed by a set of custom Macros and METS (diet and exercise plan for lifelong maintenance once you lose the weight). Regular remote check-ins with a professional can provide you with ongoing support, keep you motivated, and help you stay on track with your goals.

Finding and nurturing a support network, both online and offline, enriches your journey towards an anti-inflammatory lifestyle. It transforms this path from a solo venture into a shared experience, filled with learning, growth, and companionship. Whether through digital connections, community meetings, or personal relationships, building a support system not only strengthens your commitment but also enhances the joy and fulfillment derived from living healthily.

6.4 Celebrating Small Wins: Tracking Progress Effectively

The path to maintaining an anti-inflammatory lifestyle is often marked by small, steady steps rather than giant leaps. Recognizing and celebrating each of these steps can significantly enhance your motivation and commitment. Setting small, measurable goals that reflect your progress in tangible ways is crucial. For instance, you could set a goal to incorporate at least one anti-inflammatory superfood into your meals each day or aim to achieve a targeted wellness milestone, such as improving your digestion or reducing joint pain within a certain timeframe. These goals should be specific, achievable, relevant, and time-bound—qualities that make them clear and actionable.

Tracking your progress towards these goals can be incredibly rewarding and insightful. Various tools and apps are available to help you monitor various aspects of your health journey, from dietary intake to physical symptoms, and overall well-being. For example, food tracking apps like MyFitnessPal allow you to log your daily meals and assess your nutrient intake, ensuring you're aligning with anti-inflammatory eating principles. Other apps like Symple enable you to track symptoms and factors that influence your health, such as sleep, energy levels, and mood. By regularly reviewing this data, you can see patterns and understand what influences your inflammation—knowledge that is powerful in fine-tuning your approach.

Implementing a personal reward system can also play a pivotal role in keeping you motivated. Rewards can be a powerful incentive for maintaining your dietary and lifestyle changes. They reinforce positive behavior and celebrate achievements, no matter how small. Consider setting up a reward that you will genuinely look forward to—like a massage after a month of sticking to your anti-inflammatory meal plans, or treating yourself to a new cookbook or kitchen gadget that can help make meal preparation more enjoyable. These rewards not only celebrate your success but also encourage you to continue on your path, making the process enjoyable and something to look forward to.

Reflective practices further enhance the experience of tracking and celebrating your progress. Keeping a journal or a blog where you document your journey can be profoundly beneficial. This practice allows you to express your feelings, celebrate your successes, and articulate the challenges you face. Writing down your experiences can help you process your thoughts and reflect on your progress, providing a historical record of your journey. At any point, you can look back and see how far you've come, which can be incredibly encouraging, especially during periods when progress feels slow or when you face setbacks.

This reflective practice not only supports your emotional and mental health but also enhances your commitment to your anti-inflammatory lifestyle, reminding you of the reasons you started and the goals you are striving to achieve.

By setting clear goals, utilizing tracking tools, rewarding yourself, and engaging in reflective practices, you create a supportive framework that fosters continuous improvement and celebration of your progress. These strategies not only help keep your motivation high but also make the journey enjoyable and fulfilling. As you continue to implement these practices, remember that each small win is a stepping stone to improved health and well-being. Each positive change, each goal met, and each reflection written is a testament to your dedication and a cause for celebration.

6.5 When Results Aren't Immediate: Staying the Course

Embarking on an anti-inflammatory diet can feel like planting a garden. You prepare the soil, plant the seeds, and water diligently. Yet, despite your efforts, sprouts don't appear overnight. Similarly, when you begin integrating anti-inflammatory foods into your diet, immediate changes to your health might not be visible. It's crucial to set realistic expectations from the start. Understand that the timeline for seeing tangible benefits from dietary changes can vary greatly. Factors like your unique body chemistry, the severity of your symptoms, your overall health at the start, and how rigorously you adhere to the diet all play significant roles in the pace of your progress.

Patience and persistence are key here. Think of each anti-inflammatory meal as a step towards your goal. Staying committed can be challenging, especially when results are slow to show, but remember, gradual changes are often more sustainable and lasting. Encourage yourself by celebrating the fact that with every healthy meal, you're contributing to your body's long-term wellness. During moments of doubt, remind yourself why you started. Was it to reduce joint pain, improve digestive health, or perhaps to enhance your overall vitality? Keeping these motivations in the front of your mind can help maintain your commitment even when progress feels slow.

Periodic reassessment of your diet and lifestyle is also essential. What works for you today might not be as effective tomorrow, and that's perfectly normal. Our bodies change, our lives change, and our diets may need to evolve too. Schedule regular check-ins with yourself every few months to evaluate your progress. Are you feeling better? Are your symptoms improving? Is there something that could be adjusted for better results? This could mean tweaking your nutrient intake, introducing new anti-inflammatory foods, or even consulting with a healthcare professional for additional insights. Such adjustments are not signs of failure but are part of the dynamic process of caring for your health.

Success stories serve as powerful motivation during this ongoing process. Consider the story of Ellen, a middle-aged woman with chronic knee pain due to arthritis. After adopting an anti-inflammatory diet, it took several months before Ellen noticed a reduction in pain and an improvement in mobility. However, she didn't give up. She adjusted her diet along the way, found new recipes that excited her, and kept her goal of reducing her reliance on pain medication in sight. A year into her diet, not only had her symptoms decreased significantly, but she also enjoyed higher energy levels and better overall health. Stories like Ellen's remind us that while the effects of dietary changes can be slow to manifest, persistence can lead to substantial improvements in quality of life.

Navigating the slow pace of progress when adopting an anti-inflammatory diet requires setting realistic expectations, embracing patience, being willing to make adjustments, and drawing inspiration from the success of others. This approach not only fosters a healthier relationship with your diet but also supports a deeper, more sustainable journey to wellness. As you continue to make choices each day that align with your health goals, take comfort in knowing that each small decision contributes to a larger picture of long-term health and vitality. We want the overall goal to be the ability to live a quality life for a long time full of activity and accomplishment.

6.6 Adjusting Your Diet as Your Needs Change

As you age, undergo hormonal shifts, or experience changes in your activity levels, your dietary needs can evolve. These changes are natural and expected, and acknowledging them is crucial in maintaining your health and well-being. For instance, as you grow older, your metabolism slows down, and you might find that your body responds differently to certain foods. Hormonal changes, such as those during menopause or andropause, can also significantly impact how your body processes food and manages inflammation. Similarly, an increase in physical activity necessitates more calories and nutrients to fuel and recover from your workouts. In each case, what worked for you yesterday might not be as effective today, necessitating adjustments to your anti-inflammatory diet to align with your body's current needs.

Continuous learning and adaptation are key to successfully managing these changes. The field of nutrition, particularly related to inflammation, is constantly evolving with new research and recommendations emerging regularly. Staying informed about these developments can help you make educated decisions about your diet. For example, recent studies might highlight the benefits of a newly discovered nutrient or offer a new perspective on the best sources of antioxidants. By keeping yourself educated, you not only become proactive in your health management but also ensure that your dietary choices are supported by the latest scientific findings.

Adopting a flexible mindset towards your diet is equally important. Viewing dietary adjustments as a natural part of your health journey allows you to embrace changes without frustration. This flexibility enables you to experiment with new foods and dietary patterns that can enhance your health without feeling bound to a rigid set of rules. For example, if you find that your body responds well to a new anti-inflammatory food, such as chia seeds, incorporating them more regularly can be a delightful discovery that boosts your health. Conversely, if an old favorite no longer serves you as well as it once did, allowing yourself to let go and find alternatives can open up new dietary horizons.

Navigating life's changes with an adaptive diet, continuous learning, professional guidance if needed, and a flexible approach ensures that your anti-inflammatory eating plan remains effective and enjoyable. This proactive, responsive strategy not only supports your physical health but also enhances your relationship with food, making it a nourishing and positive aspect of your life. Together, let's banish shame being associated with food.

Reflecting on Adjusting Your Diet

In this chapter, we've explored the importance of recognizing and adapting to changes in your dietary needs as you age, experience hormonal shifts, or change activity levels. We've discussed the importance of staying informed about the latest nutrition research, regularly consulting with healthcare professionals, and maintaining a flexible approach to dietary adjustments. These strategies are crucial for ensuring that your anti-inflammatory diet continues to support your health, regardless of the changes life may bring.

As we close this chapter, remember that your diet is not just about managing inflammation—it's about supporting your life's evolving needs and enhancing your overall well-being. Embrace each change as an opportunity to refine your diet and discover what best supports your health at every stage of life.

CHAPTER 7
Success Stories and Real-life Applications

This chapter is dedicated to stories of patients who, just like you, have embraced the path of an anti-inflammatory lifestyle and witnessed profound changes in their lives. These narratives are not just tales of health regained but are testaments to the resilience of the human spirit and the power of informed choices. Each story is a beacon that lights up the path for others, showcasing the tangible benefits of dietary and lifestyle adjustments.

7.1 From Pain to Power: A Baby Boomer's Journey

Chronic Pain Management

Meet Michael, a retired school teacher and a proud grandfather, who once grappled daily with the debilitating effects of chronic joint pain. His journey began on a chilly autumn morning when the simple act of getting out of bed became a feat of will.

Diagnosed with osteoarthritis, Michael felt his independence ebbing away as his days became governed by pain medications that offered little relief and numerous side effects. The turning point came when his daughter, concerned about his worsening health, introduced him to an anti-inflammatory diet. Skeptical but desperate for a change, Michael decided to give this new approach a chance, not realizing that it would radically transform his life.

Lifestyle Adjustments

Michael's transition to an anti-inflammatory diet was gradual but deliberate. With the help of his daughter, he began to replace processed foods with whole, nutrient-rich alternatives. Meals became colorful mosaics of fruits, vegetables, lean proteins, and whole grains. Turmeric, ginger, and omega-3-rich foods like salmon became staples in his kitchen. However, the journey was not without its challenges. Michael missed his old comfort foods, and the initial phase was marked by cravings and doubts. What kept him on track was the support from his family and the small, yet noticeable, improvements in his pain levels and mobility.

Long-Term Impact

Over months, Michael experienced a significant reduction in joint pain and found himself relying less on medications. More importantly, he reclaimed the joys of his daily life. Gardening, a beloved hobby previously marred by pain, became a source of pleasure again. He could play with his grandchildren in the backyard, share in their adventures, and enjoy the simple delight of a family meal without the overshadowing presence of pain. These changes were not just physical; Michael felt a renewed sense of hope and vitality, which he attributed to his new lifestyle.

Advice to Peers

To those of his generation contemplating a similar change, Michael offers this advice: "Start small and be patient. The benefits of an anti-inflammatory diet unfold over time. It's not just about relieving pain—it's about enhancing your quality of life." He encourages finding a support system, whether it's family or a community group, to help navigate the initial hurdles and celebrate the victories. Most importantly, he suggests focusing on the foods you can add to your diet rather than those you should eliminate. This positive mindset, he found, makes the transition not only easier but also more enjoyable.

Michael's story is a powerful reminder of how lifestyle and dietary changes can dramatically enhance one's health and quality of life. It illustrates that no matter your age or the challenges you face, transformation is possible and often just a few deliberate choices away. Michael's journey from pain to power underscores the profound impact of dietary choices on our physical well-being and the broader spectrum of our lives.

7.2 A Generation X's Path to Increased Energy and Less Pain

Imagine Lisa, a vibrant Generation X professional, and mother, who once found herself plagued with persistent fatigue and nagging joint pain, both common yet debilitating issues that many face but few manage to overcome successfully. Her initial skepticism about the impact of diet on her energy levels and discomfort began to wane after a friend shared a similar story of transformation. Motivated by this, Lisa embarked on a transformative path that not only altered her diet but reshaped her entire lifestyle, bringing a newfound vigor and significantly reducing her discomfort.

Lisa's journey began with the fundamental step of overhauling her dietary habits, which primarily involved reducing processed foods and increasing her intake of anti-inflammatory ingredients. Foods rich in omega-3 fatty acids, such as salmon and flaxseeds, became staples in her kitchen, replacing the red meats and processed foods that dominated her meals. The inclusion of vibrant fruits and leafy greens not only added color to her plate but brought a variety of essential nutrients that fought against inflammation. However, dietary changes alone did not bring the rejuvenation Lisa hoped for; it was the integration of a targeted exercise regimen that began to turn the tide against her fatigue and pain.

Recognizing the synergy between diet and exercise, Lisa took up yoga and light jogging, activities chosen for their dual benefits of enhancing cardiovascular health and supporting joint mobility. This combination of anti-inflammatory eating and regular, moderate exercise created a powerful duo that tackled her pain from two angles. As her body received the nutrients it needed to fight inflammation and her muscles and joints grew stronger and more flexible, Lisa noticed a significant uplift in her energy levels and a decrease in her daily discomfort.

Family plays a pivotal role in any lifestyle overhaul, and for Lisa, this was no different. Her journey was a family affair from the beginning, with her spouse and children embracing the dietary changes alongside her. Meals became a collaborative, creative activity that not only improved Lisa's health but also brought the family closer together. They explored new recipes, learned about nutrition, and enjoyed the benefits of healthy eating as a unit. This shared experience not only made the transition smoother for Lisa but also instilled healthy habits in the entire family, creating a supportive home environment conducive to lasting change.

Professional guidance was instrumental in fine-tuning Lisa's approach to ensure her efforts were as effective as possible. Initially overwhelmed by the plethora of dietary advice available, Lisa sought the help of Lifetime Metabolic Center. This collaboration allowed her to customize her food choices to her specific health needs and preferences, ensuring her diet was both enjoyable and beneficial. Regular consultations helped Lisa stay on track, make necessary adjustments, and continuously refine her approach based on her evolving health status and goals.

Lisa's story is a compelling example of how integrating dietary changes with exercise and leveraging professional advice can dramatically enhance energy levels and reduce pain. Her experience illustrates the profound impact of a holistic approach to health and the transformative power of adopting an anti-inflammatory lifestyle. For those in Generation X, struggling with the challenges of balancing personal health with professional and family responsibilities, Lisa's story provides not just inspiration but a blueprint for rejuvenating one's health and vitality.

7.3 A Xennial's Success: Balancing Diet, Work, and Family

Navigating the demands of a bustling career and a vibrant family life, Mary, a dedicated IT manager and mother of two, found herself in a relentless cycle of stress and poor eating habits. Fast food lunches and late-night project sessions fueled by sugary snacks had become her norm, a lifestyle dictated by tight deadlines and even tighter schedules. However, the toll on her health became undeniable when she started experiencing persistent fatigue and digestive discomfort, symptoms that made her daily responsibilities feel even more burdensome. The realization that she needed a change was swift, and her decision to adopt an anti-inflammatory diet marked the beginning of a transformative chapter in her life.

Mary's approach to integrating this new dietary regimen into her already-packed schedule was methodical and thoughtful. She knew that the key to success lay in efficient meal planning and preparation. Sundays became her meal prep days, a ritual that involved the whole family. Together, they would prepare batches of anti-inflammatory meals for the week, from vibrant salads and hearty soups to grilled vegetables and lean proteins. This not only ensured that Mary had access to healthy meals during her hectic workdays but also introduced her children to the joys and benefits of nutritious eating. Quick, healthful meal ideas became a cornerstone of their family life, with smoothies packed with spinach, berries, and flaxseed for breakfast and turmeric-spiced chicken wraps for lunch. Snacks were no longer bags of chips or candy bars; instead, hummus with carrot sticks or a handful of almonds became her go-to.

This shift in dietary habits brought about a significant improvement in Mary's health. Her energy levels increased noticeably, allowing her to engage more actively with her projects at work and her family at home. More importantly, the digestive issues that once plagued her days began to diminish, a change she attributed to the anti-inflammatory properties of her new diet. But the benefits extended beyond Mary; her family too began to experience better health. Her husband, who initially joined the meal prep sessions reluctantly, found himself enjoying both the process and the meals. He lost the extra weight he had struggled with for years, and their children, previously fussy eaters, now delighted in discovering new flavors and textures. The family's eating habits transformed, fostering not only healthier bodies but also a deeper connection among them, united by the shared experience of nurturing their health.

Effective time management was crucial in Mary's ability to maintain these changes without becoming overwhelmed. She learned to prioritize tasks and delegate both at work and home, skills that allowed her to carve out time for meal planning and preparation without compromising her professional responsibilities or family time. Tools like digital calendars and meal planning apps helped keep her on track, reminding her of grocery shopping lists or when to start prepping for dinner. She also found that being upfront with her colleagues about her dietary changes and scheduling boundaries helped in managing expectations and respecting her meal times, which often included stepping away from her desk to enjoy a balanced lunch.

Mary's story is a testament to the power of taking charge of one's diet and lifestyle, even amidst the demands of a busy career and family life. Her journey underscores the importance of preparation, family involvement, and effective time management in transforming health through diet. For those facing similar challenges, her experience offers not just inspiration but practical strategies that can be adapted to fit different lifestyles, proving that with the right approach, balance is achievable, fostering not only personal health but also enriching family dynamics.

7.4 Overcoming Severe Inflammation: Stories of Hope and Health

The physical challenges of dealing with severe inflammatory conditions like rheumatoid arthritis or intense digestive disorders are profound, but the path to recovery can also bring deep, life-changing revelations. Through the narratives of individuals who have battled these severe conditions, we see the critical role an anti-inflammatory diet can play, not just in managing symptoms but in transforming lives.

For instance, consider the story of Brittany, a vibrant artist whose life was upended by the diagnosis of rheumatoid arthritis. The pain and stiffness in her joints became so severe that holding a paintbrush felt like an insurmountable task. Traditional medications provided relief but came with side effects that only added to her troubles. The breakthrough came when her rheumatologist suggested integrating an anti-inflammatory diet into her treatment plan. Skeptical at first, Brittany began eliminating processed foods and incorporating more natural, anti-inflammatory ingredients like leafy greens, nuts, and fatty fish. The change wasn't immediate, but gradually, Brittany noticed a decrease in her joint swelling and an increase in mobility that she hadn't felt in years.

Medical supervision was crucial throughout Brittany's journey. Her healthcare providers closely monitored her progress, adjusting her medications as her symptoms improved with her dietary changes. This integrated approach not only ensured her safety but also optimized her treatment, illustrating the importance of professional oversight in managing severe conditions. Her rheumatologist worked in tandem with LMC, providing Brittany with a tailored eating plan that addressed her specific nutritional needs and preferences, enhancing her overall adherence and success.

The psychological impact of dealing with severe inflammation can be as debilitating as the physical symptoms. Chronic pain and the accompanying lifestyle limitations often lead to feelings of frustration, isolation, and depression. For Brittany, the initial improvements in her physical symptoms brought about by her dietary changes had a profound positive effect on her mental health. Each small victory, each day with reduced pain, kindled a sense of hope and restored a part of her identity that had been overshadowed by her condition. This renewed optimism was crucial in motivating her to stick with her dietary changes and actively participate in her treatment and recovery.

Community support also played a pivotal role in Brittany's journey. She joined online forums and local support groups for individuals with rheumatoid arthritis, where she shared her experiences and learned from others who were on similar paths. These communities provided not only practical advice on managing symptoms and making dietary adjustments but also emotional support that helped her cope with her condition. The connections she formed proved invaluable, offering her encouragement on tough days and celebrating her successes alongside her. These interactions underscored the power of shared experiences and the comfort that comes from knowing you are not alone in your struggles.

Brittany's story, like those of many others facing severe inflammatory conditions, highlights the transformative potential of an anti-inflammatory diet when combined with medical supervision, psychological resilience, and community support. It serves as a beacon of hope for those navigating the complexities of such conditions, demonstrating that with the right approach and support, reclaiming one's health and vitality is within reach.

7.5 Professional Insights: How Dietitians Incorporate Anti-Inflammatory Principles

In the evolving field of nutrition, the role of dietitians and nutritionists is pivotal, especially when integrating anti-inflammatory principles into dietary practices. These professionals, armed with a deep understanding of the biochemical impact of foods, guide individuals through the complexities of adopting diets that can significantly mitigate inflammation-related conditions. Their expert opinions are grounded in scientific research and clinical experiences that underscore the multifaceted benefits of anti-inflammatory eating. For instance, a diet rich in omega-3 fatty acids, antioxidants, and phytonutrients has been shown to reduce markers of inflammation in the blood, such as C-reactive protein (CRP) and interleukin-6 (IL-6), which are often elevated in conditions like rheumatoid arthritis and heart disease. By reducing these markers, individuals can experience relief from pain and other symptoms associated with chronic inflammation.

Dietitians often employ case studies from their clinical practice to illustrate the effectiveness of anti-inflammatory diets. One such example involves a middle-aged woman suffering from chronic inflammatory bowel disease (IBD). Traditional medications had provided minimal relief and were accompanied by undesirable side effects. Under the guidance of a dietitian, she adopted an anti-inflammatory diet that eliminated potential food triggers like gluten and processed sugars while incorporating healing foods like bone broth and fermented vegetables. Over several months, her symptoms improved significantly, allowing her to reduce her medication dosage under medical supervision. This case not only highlights the potential of dietary changes to complement medical treatment but also emphasizes the importance of personalized dietary strategies.

Customization of dietary plans is a cornerstone of effective nutrition therapy, particularly when dealing with inflammation. Dietitians consider various factors such as individual allergies, food preferences, and existing health conditions to tailor dietary recommendations that are both effective and sustainable. For someone with celiac disease and chronic joint pain, a dietitian might recommend a gluten-free, anti-inflammatory diet that includes specific supplements like turmeric and fish oil to address both the autoimmune and inflammatory components of the patient's conditions. This approach ensures that dietary interventions are not only targeted and effective but also adaptable to an individual's lifestyle and needs.

Continuous education and adaptation are essential in the field of nutrition, especially given the rapid pace of research in dietary inflammation. Professionals remain abreast of the latest studies and emerging food science to refine their recommendations and provide the most up-to-date advice to their clients. This commitment to ongoing education is crucial, not only for enhancing the knowledge and skills of the dietitians themselves but also for ensuring that patients receive the most effective and scientifically supported care available. Moreover, this continuous learning process often includes attending conferences, participating in workshops, and subscribing to leading nutrition journals, activities that help professionals stay at the cutting edge of nutritional science.

As dietitians integrate these anti-inflammatory principles into their practice, they not only change the diets of individuals but also influence the broader understanding of how deeply our food choices impact our health. Through their expert guidance, tailored approaches, and commitment to education, these professionals play a crucial role in fostering a healthier society where dietary choices are seen as integral to managing and preventing chronic diseases. This holistic approach to nutrition, grounded in the understanding and application of anti-inflammatory principles, continues to empower countless individuals to take control of their health and lead fuller, more vibrant lives.

7.6 The Role of Community in Sustaining Lifestyle Changes

The benefits of being part of a community are fantastic, providing not just motivation and accountability, but also a plethora of shared knowledge and experiences. You're not just changing your diet; you're joining a collective journey of hundreds, perhaps thousands, who are on the same path, each with unique insights and advice.

Let's explore the successful models of community support which have proven effective. Local wellness groups, often found in community centers or even through healthcare providers, offer regular meetings where individuals can share their experiences, challenges, and successes. These groups often feature educational components, with nutritionists or doctors speaking on relevant topics, and provide a platform for members to ask questions and receive guidance. Online forums and social media groups dedicated to anti-inflammatory lifestyles serve a similar purpose but with the added convenience of accessibility. Platforms like Facebook and specialized health forums mentioned earlier are bustling with active communities where members exchange recipes, tips for managing flare-ups, and words of encouragement. These digital gatherings can be particularly valuable for those who may not have access to local groups or who prefer the anonymity that online interactions can offer.

Building your support network is another crucial element in sustaining your dietary changes. Engaging family, friends, and colleagues about your new lifestyle can open doors to unexpected support. Start by sharing your reasons for adopting an anti-inflammatory diet and the benefits you hope to gain or have already experienced. This not only educates your loved ones but can also invite them to support you more actively. Perhaps a family member will also be inspired to join you, or a friend can share their own experiences with dietary changes. At work, communicating your dietary needs can lead to considerations during catered meetings or office parties, ensuring there are options available that align with your dietary choices.

Maintaining long-term engagement with your community is crucial for ongoing support and motivation. Regular participation in community events, whether online webinars, local workshops, or group discussions, keeps the connection active and provides continual learning opportunities. Sharing your successes and setbacks not only contributes to the pool of collective knowledge but also helps you reflect on your journey. This exchange of stories can be profoundly motivating, not just for you but also for others in the community who may be struggling or seeking encouragement. Additionally, contributing to discussions, whether by answering a newcomer's questions or by offering tips on overcoming common challenges, can reinforce your knowledge and commitment to your anti-inflammatory lifestyle.

As we wrap up this chapter on the pivotal role of community in maintaining anti-inflammatory lifestyle changes, it's clear that the journey is as much about connecting with others as it is about changing your diet. The shared experiences, the collective wisdom, and the mutual support found in community interactions enrich your journey, making the path less daunting and more enjoyable. As we move forward, remember that each step you take not only brings you closer to your own health goals but also contributes to a larger tapestry of communal health and well-being.

In the next chapter, we will explore advanced topics in managing inflammation, offering you deeper insights and broader perspectives on how to fine-tune your lifestyle to combat chronic inflammation more effectively. This will include cutting-edge research, innovative treatments, and emerging trends that will equip you with the knowledge to continue refining your approach.

CHAPTER 8
Advanced Topics in Anti-Inflammatory Practices

Take a deep breath, sit upright in your chair, and imagine you are a seasoned gardener, stepping into a greenhouse full of exotic herbs and spices, each with its own unique fragrance and set of powerful healing properties. Smell the smells, feel the breezes, and reset your mind and body. This chapter offers you an opportunity to delve deeper into the world of anti-inflammatory herbs and spices. As you explore this garden, you'll uncover the rich tapestry of benefits these natural wonders can bring to your life, not just for their flavor, but for their profound health benefits. Let's embark on this exploration together, discovering how these ancient remedies can be seamlessly integrated into your modern life to combat inflammation and enhance your well-being.

8.1 Anti-Inflammatory Herbs and Spices: Deep Dive into Uses and Benefits

Turmeric, ginger, garlic, and cinnamon are not just culinary delights; they are storied herbs and spices with deep roots in traditional medicine across various cultures. Known for their potent anti-inflammatory properties, these ingredients are powerhouses in combating inflammation and enhancing overall health. Each of these herbs and spices contains active compounds that interact with your body in unique ways to reduce inflammation and promote healing.

Turmeric is perhaps one of the most celebrated anti-inflammatory herbs, widely recognized for its bright yellow color and robust flavor. The active compound in turmeric, curcumin, has been extensively studied for its anti-inflammatory effects. Curcumin works by blocking NF-kB, a molecule that travels into the nuclei of your cells and turns on genes related to inflammation. NF-kB is believed to play a major role in many chronic diseases. Incorporating turmeric into your diet can be as simple as adding a teaspoon to your morning smoothie or sprinkling it over roasted vegetables, lending a warm, peppery flavor.

Ginger, with its zesty and pungent profile, is another formidable anti-inflammatory agent. Gingerols, the main bioactive compound in ginger, have been shown to have anti-inflammatory and antioxidant effects. This spice can help reduce muscle pain and soreness, and it has been used to ease nausea and digestive issues for centuries. Ginger can be used fresh, dried, or as an oil or juice. It's a versatile ingredient that can be added to stir-fries, steeped into a soothing tea, or blended into dressings and sauces.

Garlic, with its unmistakable aroma and taste, is not only a staple in cuisine worldwide but also packed with health benefits. It contains compounds such as allicin, which have been found to reduce inflammation and offer antioxidant benefits. Regular consumption of garlic can help combat sickness, including the common cold, by boosting the immune system. Garlic is incredibly easy to incorporate into your diet; it can be added to almost any savory dish for an extra layer of flavor.

Cinnamon is not just for desserts. This sweet and woody spice contains cinnamaldehyde, which has anti-inflammatory properties. It can help lower blood sugar levels, reduce heart disease risk factors, and has a boatload of other impressive health benefits. Sprinkling cinnamon on your oatmeal, adding it to your coffee or tea, or using it in your baking are great ways to enjoy its benefits daily.

To bring these spices into your daily routine, consider starting your day with a cup of **golden milk**, a traditional Indian drink that involves simmering milk (dairy or plant-based) with turmeric and other spices like cinnamon and ginger. Another therapeutic recipe is **ginger-infused tea**, which can be made by steeping fresh ginger in boiling water, a perfect remedy for soothing inflammation after meals.

Recent scientific research continues to support the health benefits of these herbs and spices. Studies have shown that regular consumption of these ingredients can significantly reduce markers of inflammation in the body. For instance, a study published in the Journal of Medicinal Food found that turmeric extract supplements significantly reduced inflammation in patients with arthritis.

In this verdant garden of nature's own medicine, you have the power to transform your health through the simple act of seasoning your meals. Each sprinkle of cinnamon, each clove of garlic, each slice of ginger, and each pinch of turmeric you incorporate into your regular diet, offers not just a burst of flavor but a boost of anti-inflammatory power. As you continue to explore these spices and integrate them into your meals, remember that each small step you take is a leap toward being the healthiest you.

8.2 The Science of Omega-3s and Their Role in Anti-Inflammation

As mentioned several places here already, Omega-3 fatty acids are like the unsung heroes of your cellular health, especially when it comes to inflammation. These fats are not just another nutritional component; they are pivotal in modulating inflammatory processes within your body. Omega-3s primarily exert their effects through the production of substances called eicosanoids, which have potent effects on inflammation and your immune system. Eicosanoids made from omega-3 fatty acids are often anti-inflammatory, helping to reduce the production of inflammatory cytokines and eicosanoids that are derived from other types of fatty acids. This biochemical role is crucial, as chronic inflammation is linked to a range of conditions from heart disease to arthritis, and managing it can lead to significant improvements in health and well-being.

You can find these beneficial omega-3s in a variety of foods, and they're commonly categorized into three types: ALA (alpha-linolenic acid), found in plant oils like flaxseed, walnuts, and chia seeds; and EPA (eicosapentaenoic acid) and DHA (docosahexaenoic acid), which are primarily found in marine oils like those from fish and algae. ALA is an essential fat, meaning your body can't produce it, so it must be consumed in your diet. It serves as a building block that can be converted in small amounts to EPA and DHA in the body, though this process isn't very efficient. EPA and DHA, on the other hand, are ready to use and don't require transformation by the body, which makes them highly effective. They are particularly influential in brain health and reducing inflammatory responses.

When considering the inclusion of omega-3 supplements in your diet, it's important to choose high-quality products to ensure purity and effectiveness. Fish oil is the most common source of omega-3 supplements and can vary widely in terms of concentration and purity. It's advisable to look for supplements that have been certified by third parties for safety and quality, and those that are sourced sustainably to protect ocean biodiversity. The recommended dosage can vary depending on your specific health conditions and goals, but generally, a daily intake of 250-500 mg of combined EPA and DHA is often recommended for healthy adults. For those dealing with health issues related to inflammation, higher dosages may be beneficial and should be discussed with a healthcare provider.

Clinical studies have robustly documented the benefits of omega-3s in managing chronic inflammatory diseases. For instance, research has demonstrated that omega-3 fatty acid supplements can significantly reduce the pain and stiffness associated with rheumatoid arthritis, an autoimmune disease characterized by significant inflammation. Similarly, studies on heart disease have shown that omega-3s can reduce the incidence of cardiovascular events, like heart attacks, partly due to their anti-inflammatory effects. These findings not only reinforce the importance of omega-3s in a healthy diet but also highlight their potential as a therapeutic agent in managing and potentially preventing chronic diseases driven by inflammation. A few recently released articles appear to question this science, but upon further inspection, they mainly stress the importance of quality.

Incorporating omega-3s into your diet isn't just about taking supplements; it's about making deliberate choices to include anti-inflammatory foods that can transform your health. Whether you choose to sprinkle chia seeds on your breakfast, enjoy a salmon steak for dinner, or take a high-quality fish oil supplement, these small choices can lead to big changes in your inflammatory status and overall health. As you continue to explore the impact of nutrition on inflammation, remember that these powerful fats are more than just a supplement; they are a key part of a holistic approach to a healthier, vibrant life.

8.3 Advanced Meal-Prepping Techniques for Dietary Success Recapped

As briefly touched upon earlier, stepping into the kitchen, equipped with a plan and the right tools, can transform meal preparation from a daily chore into a powerful strategy to maintain your anti-inflammatory diet. One of the keys to successful meal prepping is efficiency—maximizing your time and efforts in the kitchen to ensure you have healthy, delicious meals ready when you need them. Embrace the concept of multitasking while cooking. For instance, while a pot of quinoa is simmering, you could be roasting vegetables in the oven and blending a batch of a ginger-turmeric dressing in your blender. Utilizing kitchen gadgets like slow cookers and pressure cookers can also be a game-changer. These tools allow you to prepare components of your meals or entire dishes with minimal active cooking time, letting you set them up and continue with your day while they cook. This approach not only saves time but also helps in preparing large batches of meals, crucial for sticking to your diet throughout the week.

Preserving the nutrients in your food during meal prep is just as important as the cooking itself. Techniques such as proper chopping—using sharp knives to make clean cuts—help in retaining the integrity and nutritional value of fresh produce.

Cooking methods also play a pivotal role; steaming or lightly sautéing vegetables preserves more vitamins and minerals compared to long cooking processes. Similarly, the use of acid, like a squeeze of lemon juice over cut fruits or avocados, can prevent oxidation and preserve the nutritional content and appearance of fresh ingredients. When it comes to storing, keep your cooked meals and prepped ingredients in air-tight containers in the refrigerator or freezer to maintain their freshness and prevent spoilage. These practices ensure that each meal you prepare is not only rich in flavor but also maximizes the anti-inflammatory benefits of the ingredients.

Theme-based meal prep can inject fun and variety into your diet, making it more enjoyable and sustainable. Consider designating themes for different days of the week, such as Mediterranean Mondays or Thai Tuesdays, which can help in planning and looking forward to your meals. Each theme can focus on incorporating specific anti-inflammatory ingredients prevalent in those cuisines, like olive oil and leafy greens for Mediterranean recipes, or turmeric and ginger for Thai dishes. This approach not only simplifies shopping and preparation but also ensures a diverse intake of nutrients and flavors throughout the week, keeping your diet balanced and exciting.

When it comes to feeding a family, meal prepping can seem daunting, especially when considering everyone's tastes and dietary needs. However, strategies like scaling recipes and customizing meal components can make it manageable. Prepare base ingredients, such as grilled chicken or roasted vegetables, in large quantities, and then vary the spices or accompanying sides to cater to different family members' preferences. For instance, you might serve a simple grilled chicken with pasta for the kids, while adding a spicy salsa for adults. Encouraging family members to participate in meal prep can also help in accommodating individual preferences and makes it an engaging activity that everyone can look forward to. This not only ensures that the meals meet the dietary needs of all family members but also fosters a shared commitment to healthy eating, reinforcing the anti-inflammatory diet as a family-wide lifestyle choice.

8.4 Combating Autoimmune Conditions with Diet: What the Latest Research Shows

Understanding the complex relationship between diet and autoimmune conditions is akin to unraveling a tightly woven tapestry. Each thread represents different factors like gut health and food sensitivities, which when pulled correctly, can help manage or even alleviate symptoms of autoimmune diseases. Our gut health, notably, plays a pivotal role in our overall immune function. The gut is not only a digestive organ but an immune center, housing a vast majority of our immune cells. When the gut's delicate balance is disrupted, it can trigger an immune response that may exacerbate or potentially trigger autoimmune conditions. Foods that irritate the gut or cause an imbalance in gut bacteria can lead to increased gut permeability, often referred to as 'leaky gut'. This condition allows particles that are not typically bioavailable to enter the bloodstream, potentially leading to an autoimmune response.

In addressing these challenges, the Autoimmune Protocol (AIP) diet has emerged as a therapeutic tool for many. This diet goes beyond standard dietary recommendations by eliminating food groups that are potential irritants to the gut and immune system, such as grains, legumes, nuts, seeds, nightshade vegetables, and dairy. The focus is on consuming nutrient-dense foods that heal and restore gut health, including organ meats, starchy vegetables, fermented foods, and bone broth. The AIP diet is designed to reduce inflammation and heal autoimmune conditions by resetting the immune system and reducing gut inflammation that might be driving the disease process.

Emerging research continues to shed light on new dietary strategies and foods that could benefit individuals with autoimmune conditions. Recent studies have highlighted the potential of certain polyphenols found in fruits and vegetables to modulate immune function and reduce inflammation. Additionally, advancements in understanding the microbiome are leading to more targeted approaches in diet therapy for autoimmune diseases, focusing on prebiotics and probiotics to restore gut health. These insights not only deepen our understanding of how diet influences autoimmunity but also pave the way for new treatments that are more aligned with the natural demands of our bodies. As we continue to explore and understand these connections, the potential to significantly alter the course of autoimmune diseases through diet becomes a tangible reality. Through careful consideration and application of these dietary strategies, you have the power to take control of your health and potentially transform your life in profound ways.

8.5 The Future of Anti-Inflammatory Eating: Trends and Innovations

As we stand at the cusp of daily, minute-by-minute technological advancement, the realm of anti-inflammatory eating is poised to undergo transformative shifts that promise to reshape our approach to health and wellness. The integration of personalized nutrition apps and AI-driven diet planning tools marks a significant leap forward. Imagine an app that analyzes your dietary needs based on genetic makeup, lifestyle, and health goals, then tailors a meal plan specifically designed to reduce inflammation in your body. These smart technologies utilize complex algorithms to process vast amounts of data, offering recommendations that are not only precise but also adaptable to your changing health needs. Such innovations make the journey towards an anti-inflammatory lifestyle more accessible, providing you with insights and adjustments that are as dynamic as your life.

Sustainability in diet is another frontier where significant strides are being made. The connection between what you eat and where your food comes from has profound implications on both health and environmental impact. By choosing locally sourced, organic foods, you not only reduce the consumption of harmful pesticides and chemicals but also support sustainable farming practices that contribute to the health of our planet. This conscious choice to embrace locally grown produce ensures that the foods you consume are fresher, packed with more nutrients, and have a lower carbon footprint due to reduced transportation distances. As communities continue to grow more aware of these benefits, we see a burgeoning trend towards diets that prioritize environmental sustainability alongside personal health, creating a harmonious balance that nurtures both the individual and the world they inhabit.

In the arena of food innovation, researchers and food scientists are tirelessly working to develop products that specifically target inflammation. Imagine walking down a grocery aisle and picking up foods enriched with specialized probiotic strains designed to enhance gut health and reduce inflammatory responses. Or consider the potential of plant-based compounds engineered to mimic the anti-inflammatory effects of medications but without the side effects. These innovative products are not just conceptual but are becoming realities as more companies invest in foods that support a holistic approach to health. This shift towards functional foods, which not only nourish but also heal, is a testament to the growing recognition of diet as a cornerstone of health management.

Looking ahead, the landscape of anti-inflammatory diets is expected to evolve with an increasing emphasis on personalization and prevention. As global health trends lean more towards proactive rather than reactive measures, the demand for diets that can prevent inflammation and associated diseases is likely to rise. This shift is supported by a growing body of research that underscores the role of diet in maintaining long-term health and preventing chronic illnesses. With advancements in technology and a deeper understanding of nutritional science, we are on the brink of a new era where diet is tailored not just to the diseases we aim to cure but to the prevention of those diseases before they arise.

In this dynamic and evolving landscape, your role as an informed individual is more crucial than ever. By staying abreast of these trends and innovations, you empower yourself with the knowledge to make choices that align with both your personal health goals and the broader vision of a sustainable, healthier world.

8.6 Integrating Anti-Inflammatory Eating with Other Therapeutic Diets

Navigating the landscape of dietary management, particularly when dealing with chronic conditions, often involves blending various nutritional strategies to achieve optimal health outcomes. Integrating the anti-inflammatory diet with other therapeutic diets such as the ketogenic, low-FODMAP, or Mediterranean diets can often enhance the effectiveness of your dietary approach. This synergy can be especially beneficial in addressing complex health issues where multiple bodily systems may be affected.

Each of these diets brings its own strengths to the table. For example, the ketogenic diet, which is high in fats and low in carbohydrates, has been shown to reduce inflammation through the reduction of blood sugar levels and the production of ketones that have anti-inflammatory properties. When combined with anti-inflammatory foods that are high in omega-3 fatty acids and antioxidants, the ketogenic diet can be tailored to reduce systemic inflammation. Similarly, the Mediterranean diet, which emphasizes fruits, vegetables, whole grains, and healthy fats, naturally aligns with anti-inflammatory principles. Its rich content of polyphenols and unsaturated fats can further help in reducing inflammatory markers, particularly in cardiovascular diseases.

The low-FODMAP diet, which is often used to manage gastrointestinal symptoms in conditions like IBS, restricts foods that are high in certain fermentable carbohydrates. Integrating anti-inflammatory principles into this diet involves choosing fruits and vegetables that are low in FODMAPs yet high in anti-inflammatory properties, such as ginger and turmeric, which can help manage digestive inflammation without triggering symptoms.

In a compelling case study, John, a 45-year-old with irritable bowel syndrome (IBS) and joint pain, integrated the low-FODMAP and anti-inflammatory diets under the guidance of a dietitian. By eliminating high-FODMAP foods that triggered his IBS symptoms and incorporating anti-inflammatory foods like leafy greens and fatty fish, John experienced significant relief not only in his digestive symptoms but also in his joint pain. His case illustrates the potential of diet synergy in managing co-existing conditions effectively.

When considering the integration of these dietary approaches, it's crucial to maintain nutritional balance and adequacy. This often involves careful planning to ensure that dietary restrictions from one plan do not lead to deficiencies when combined with another. For instance, while merging ketogenic and anti-inflammatory diets, one must ensure adequate fiber intake, as ketogenic diets can sometimes lack sufficient fiber due to the restriction of some fruits and vegetables.

Nutrition experts often advocate for a personalized approach when combining dietary strategies. Each individual's response to different foods can vary significantly based on genetic factors, existing health conditions, and overall lifestyle. Professionals emphasize the importance of monitoring inflammatory markers and other health indicators regularly to adjust the diet as needed. This personalized strategy ensures that the diet not only aims to alleviate symptoms but also supports holistic health and well-being.

By understanding and implementing these integrative dietary strategies, you empower yourself to navigate your health with informed choices, blending the best of various nutritional approaches to suit your unique health needs. This tailored approach not only enhances your ability to manage symptoms effectively but also supports your overall health in the long term, making your diet a powerful punch in your fight for wellness.

As we conclude this exploration of integrating anti-inflammatory eating with other therapeutic diets, remember that the essence of effective dietary management lies in its personalization and adaptability. The fusion of different dietary principles should be tailored to fit your health profile and goals, guided by professional advice, and adjusted as your needs evolve. This chapter has equipped you with the knowledge and insights to blend these dietary strategies effectively, setting the stage for you to continue building a nourishing and health-promoting eating plan. As you move forward, carry with you the understanding that your diet can be as dynamic and multifaceted as the life you lead, adapting and evolving in harmony with your health needs.

CONCLUSION

As we draw this guide to a close, I want to take a moment to reflect on the journey we've embarked on together through the pages of this book. Our primary goal was to demystify the anti-inflammatory diet, making it accessible and practical for everyone, regardless of your culinary skills or budget. We've explored the fundamentals of inflammation, the pivotal steps to starting an anti-inflammatory lifestyle, and the myriad of delicious, quick recipes that support gut health, disease prevention, and ultimately enhance your longevity.

Each chapter was crafted to provide you with the knowledge and tools to understand and manage inflammation—a condition that, if left unchecked, can affect not just your physical well-being but your overall quality of life. From the basics of inflammatory responses to comprehensive meal planning and preparation strategies, we covered essential elements that form the pillars of an anti-inflammatory lifestyle.

Remember, adopting an anti-inflammatory diet is a deeply personal journey. It's about tuning in to your body's needs and responding with nourishment that heals and revitalizes. I encourage you to take what you've learned here and tailor it to fit your unique health requirements and lifestyle preferences. Use this book as your compass, guiding you toward healthier choices, one meal at a time.

The success stories sprinkled throughout the book are testaments to the transformative power of making concerted dietary changes. These narratives are not just stories; they are experiences from patients who took control of their health and witnessed significant improvements. Let these stories inspire you as you forge your path toward a healthier life.

It's important to acknowledge that change doesn't happen overnight. Patience and persistence are your allies on this journey. Some days will be easier than others, and that's perfectly okay. What matters most is your commitment to continue, to adjust your course as needed, and to always prioritize your well-being.

For those of you who may have specific health challenges or find certain aspects of dietary change daunting, I strongly advocate consulting with a healthcare professional. Their guidance can be invaluable, providing personalized advice that ensures your dietary choices support your health goals effectively and safely.

Now, I invite you to start making small, manageable changes. Perhaps pick a recipe from Chapter 3 to try this week, or experiment with one of the meal planning techniques we discussed in Chapter 4. Every small step you take is a stride towards a healthier you.

I would love to hear about your journey. Share your experiences, challenges, and victories with me through our community at Lifelong Metabolic Center, or connect with me on social media. Your stories not only inspire others but also enrich our collective understanding of health and wellness.

Visit www.lifelongmetaboliccenter.com for continuous support, updates, and resources that can assist you in losing weight, resetting your metabolism, and/or maintaining an anti-inflammatory lifestyle. Your feedback and engagement are what drive this community forward, helping all of us learn and grow together.

Thank you for trusting me to guide you through this transformative process. It's been an honor to share this knowledge with you, and I am excited to see how you bring these practices into your life. Here's to your health, happiness, and a vibrant, inflammation-free future!

With gratitude and best wishes,

Dr. Amanda Borre, D.C.

We at LMC count on positive reviews to help pass this great information along. Please take a moment to go to amazon.com to leave us a review. Much love!!

REFERENCES

- *25 Anti-Inflammatory Breakfasts in 15 Minutes https://www.eatingwell.com/gallery/7916792/anti-inflammatory-breakfasts-in-15-minutes/*

- *9 Herbs and Spices That Fight Inflammation https://www.healthline.com/nutrition/anti-inflammatory-herbs*

- *Anti-Inflammatory Diet 101: How to Reduce Inflammation ... https://www.healthline.com/nutrition/anti-inflammatory-diet-101*

- *Anti-inflammatory food superstars for every season https://www.health.harvard.edu/blog/anti-inflammatory-food-superstars-for-every-season-202111302648*

- *Anti-Inflammatory Meal Plan for Beginners https://www.eatingwell.com/article/7894310/anti-inflammatory-meal-plan-for-beginners/*

- *Anti-Inflammatory Meal Plan: Recipes for 7 Days https://www.healthline.com/health/rheumatoid-ar-*

thritis/seven-day-meal-plan

- *Barriers and facilitators to adhering to an anti-inflammatory ... https://www.ncbi.nlm.nih.gov/pmc/articles/PMC6122254/*

- *Chronic Inflammation - StatPearls https://www.ncbi.nlm.nih.gov/books/NBK493173/*

- *Chronic Inflammation in the Context of Everyday Life https://www.ncbi.nlm.nih.gov/pmc/articles/PMC7312944/*

- *Current and Future Nutritional Strategies to Modulate ... https://www.ncbi.nlm.nih.gov/pmc/articles/PMC6718105/*

- *Diet Review: Anti-Inflammatory Diet | The Nutrition Source https://www.hsph.harvard.edu/nutrition-source/healthy-weight/diet-reviews/anti-inflammatory-diet/*

- *Diet Review: Anti-Inflammatory Diet | The Nutrition Source https://www.hsph.harvard.edu/nutrition-source/healthy-weight/diet-reviews/anti-inflammatory-diet/*

- *Do pro-inflammatory diets harm our health? And can anti- ... https://www.health.harvard.edu/blog/do-pro-inflammatory-di-*

ets-harm-our-health-and-can-anti-inflammatory-diets-help-2020122321624

- *Eating Out? How to Stick to Your Anti-Inflammatory Diet at ... https://www.rupahealth.com/post/eating-out-how-to-stick-to-your-anti-inflammatory-diet-at-restaurants*

- *Efficacy of the Autoimmune Protocol Diet for Inflammatory ... https://www.ncbi.nlm.nih.gov/pmc/articles/PMC5647120/*

- *Food, Health, and the Gen X-Factor: A Generation ... https://foodinsight.org/generation-x-consumer-habits/*

- *Foods that fight inflammation https://www.health.harvard.edu/staying-healthy/foods-that-fight-inflammation*

- *How sleep deprivation can cause inflammation https://www.health.harvard.edu/healthbeat/how-sleep-deprivation-can-cause-inflammation*

- *How to Understand and Use the Nutrition Facts Label https://www.fda.gov/food/nutrition-facts-label/how-understand-and-use-nutrition-facts-label*

- *Must have kitchen tools for healthy cooking https://www.heartandstroke.ca/articles/must-have-kitchen-*

tools-for-healthy-cooking

- *Omega-3 Fatty Acids - Health Professional Fact Sheet https://ods.od.nih.gov/factsheets/Omega3FattyAc-ids-HealthProfessional/*

- *Overcoming diet and exercise slips https://www. mdanderson.org/publications/focused-on-health/ overcoming-diet-slips.h31Z1590624.html*

- *Quick-start guide to an anti-inflammation diet https://www.health.harvard.edu/staying-healthy/ quick-start-guide-to-an-antiinflammation-diet*

- *Support groups: Make connections, get help https:// www.mayoclinic.org/healthy-lifestyle/stress-man-agement/in-depth/support-groups/art-20044655*

- *The 6 Best Budget-Friendly Anti-Inflammatory Foods ... https://www.eatingwell.com/article/8024844/ best-budget-friendly-anti-inflammatory-foods/*

- *The 6 Best Budget-Friendly Anti-Inflammatory Foods, According to a Dietitian https://www.eatingwell.com/ article/8024844/best-budget-friendly-anti-inflamma-tory-foods/*

- *The anti-inflammatory effects of exercise: mechanisms and ... https://www.nature.com/articles/nri3041*

- *The Impact of Stress on Inflammation: Coping Strate-*

gies for a Healthier Life https://www.rupahealth.com/ post/the-impact-of-stress-on-inflammation-coping-strategies-for-a-healthier-life

- *Turmeric Benefits https://www.hopkinsmedicine.org/ health/wellness-and-prevention/turmeric-benefits*

- *Unprocessed Foods Diet: Benefits, Examples, Tips https://www.health.com/nutrition/eat-clean-give-up-processed-foods*

- *Unveiling the therapeutic symphony of probiotics, prebiotics ... https://www.ncbi.nlm.nih.gov/pmc/articles/ PMC10881654/*

- *What does the evidence say about anti-inflammatory diets? https://www.medicalnewstoday.com/articles/ do-anti-inflammatory-diets-really-work*

Printed in Great Britain
by Amazon

51696773R00088